FIRST AID
FOR
CHILDREN
FAST

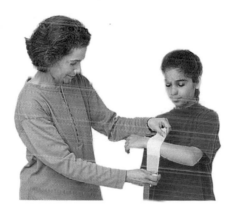

Canadian Edition

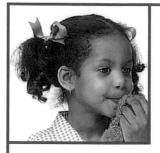
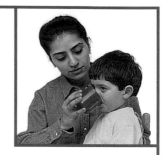

FIRST AID
FOR
CHILDREN
FAST

Canadian Consultant
Paul Munk, M.D., F.R.C.P.(C.)

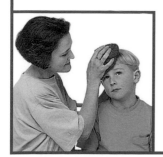
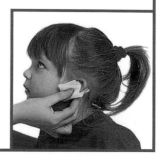

Editor Joanna Benwell
Senior Editor Janet Mohun
US Senior Editor Jill Hamilton
Art Editors Sara Freeman, Floyd Sayers
DTP Designer Julian Dams
Senior Managing Editor Jemima Dunne
Managing Art Editor Louise Dick
Production Wendy Penn
Photography Gary Ombler
Editor, Canadian Edition Julia Roles

First Canadian edition 2003

03 04 05 06/10 9 8 7 6 5 4 3 2 1

Copyright © 1994, 1999, 2002, 2003 Dorling Kindersley Limited

Dorling Kindersley is represented in Canada by
Tourmaline Editions Inc.
662 King Street West, Suite 304
Toronto, Ontario M5V 1M7

National Library of Canada Cataloguing in Publication Data
First aid for children fast /Canadian consultant, Paul Munk. -- 1st. Canadian ed.
Includes index
ISBN 1-55363-019-X
    1. Pediatric emergencies--Popular works. 2. First aid in illness and injury. I. Munk, Paul
RJ370.F58 2003   618.92'00252   C2003-900919-X

Reproduced in Italy by GRB Editrice, Verona
Printed and bound in Italy by Graphicom

Discover more at
www.dk.com

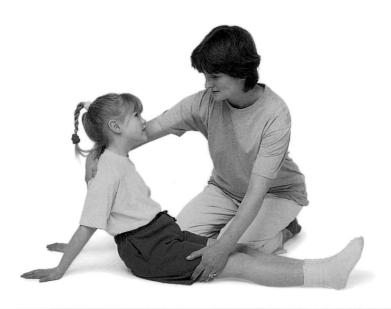

FOREWORD

Paediatrics evolved as a specialty because children aren't just small adults. Their problems require different approaches and techniques. So before emergencies occur, carers need to check out the local medical facilities – including emergency departments, walk-in clinics, and medical offices. Which ones have staff specially trained to deal with infants and children, and equipment designed specifically for their needs?

"Be prepared" is the theme of this book, and I hope it will be read before the moment of crisis – before an emergency happens. Caregivers will then have its contents at their fingertips, and can share the information with others.

As a community paediatrician in the Greater Toronto Area for the past twenty-seven years, and through my work at the Hospital for Sick Children, I've had considerable exposure to paediatric first aid. As Assistant Professor of Paediatrics at the University of Toronto, I teach these skills to students. And as a Board Member and Past President of the Canadian Paediatric Society, I've been involved with setting standards for emergency care across Canada.

I'd like to share some of this experience with you, and I hope you will use this book as a partner in reaching our common goal – the well-being of children.

Paul Munk, M.D., F.R.C.P.(C.)

Senior Staff Physician
Hospital for Sick Children, Toronto

Assistant Professor of Paediatrics
University of Toronto

CONTENTS

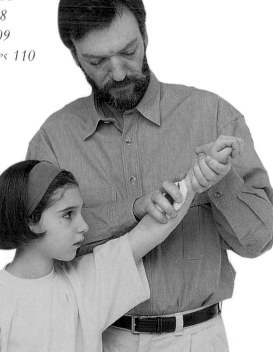

INTRODUCTION

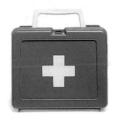 This book has been compiled primarily for parents but also for other caregivers – grandparents, daycare workers, teachers, babysitters, playgroup leaders – who may regularly, or even occasionally, find themselves in charge of infants, children, and adolescents. The content has been set out in a clear and logical way and the information presented largely in pictorial form using simple words and captions to make it very easy to follow and to understand. The first aid methods and techniques described are in accordance with accepted modern practice and are in compliance with guidelines set for paediatric advanced life support (PALS), developed by the Canadian Paediatric Society, the American Heart Association, and the American Academy of Pediatrics.

Emergencies are by their very nature unexpected events and require a prompt and proper response. If you follow the advice and guidance given in this book you will be able to give early and effective help whenever it is needed. You should be aware, however, that first aid is essentially a practical skill and your confidence and effectiveness will be greatly enhanced by expert training in a practical setting. St. John Ambulance Canada and the Canadian Red Cross have chapters throughout the country and regularly run a wide variety of first aid and cardiopulmonary resuscitation courses, some exclusively concerned with first aid for infants and children. You can find out more about these by calling your local branches or checking their web sites.

Giving first aid – coping with the emergency and doing the right thing promptly and effectively – can be straightforward but it can also be stressful, sometimes distasteful (especially if the child is not your own), and even dangerous. It is important that you remain in control of your feelings and avoid any tendency to an impulsive, rash action that could result in additional harm to an injured child or to yourself. You cannot give effective help if you yourself become a victim, so you must always take a little time to think before you act. This book is intended to help you do the right thing at the right time – safely and effectively.

How to use this book

This book covers first aid treatment for everything from minor cuts and scrapes to resuscitation. For every condition a series of photographs shows you exactly what to do in an emergency. Key pieces of information are indicated on the photographs and supplementary advice can be found alongside in the step-by-step text.

The injuries are organized by type, in sections such as WOUNDS AND BLEEDING and BITES AND STINGS. However, in an emergency, the thumbnail index on the back cover will direct you right to the relevant page.

There are also sections such as ACTION IN AN EMERGENCY and BANDAGES AND DRESSINGS, that contain information for general reference.

Key signs and symptoms help you recognize the conditions

Clear photographs illustrate every step of treatment

Annotations highlight essential action

The quick reference index on the back cover gives instant access to major first aid emergencies

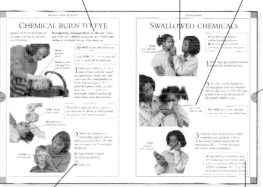

Symbols highlight the action necessary for further medical attention

Cross-references direct you to other pages where information is given about associated injuries

Guide to the symbols
The following symbols and instructions appear if your child needs further medical attention:

ⓒ CALL A DOCTOR
(Telephone for further advice.)

✚ TAKE YOUR CHILD TO THE HOSPITAL
(Your child needs to be seen in the emergency department.)

☎ CALL 911
(Your child needs urgent medical attention and is best transported to the hospital by ambulance.)

☠ CALL YOUR LOCAL POISON CONTROL CENTER OR 1-800-268-9017 for information on poisons.

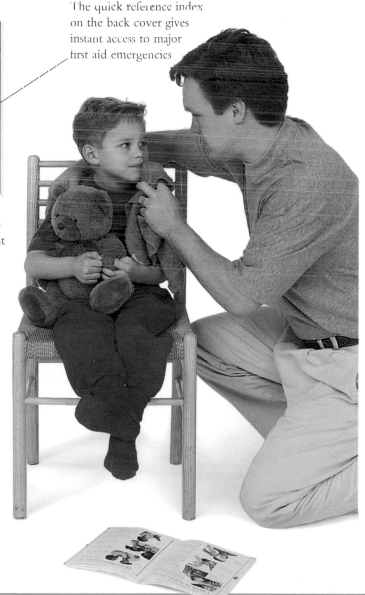

9

ACTION IN AN EMERGENCY

In any emergency, particularly one involving children, it is important to keep calm and act logically. Remember four steps:

1 Assess the situation

- What happened?
- How did it happen?
- Is there more than one injured child?
- Is there any continuing danger?
- Is there anyone who can help?
- Do I need an ambulance?

2 Think of safety

- Do not risk injuring yourself – you cannot help if you become a victim
- Remove any source of danger from your child
- Move your child only if you must and do so very carefully

3 Treat serious injuries first

In children, there are two conditions that immediately threaten life:
- *Inability to breathe* (see ABC OF RESUSCITATION, p.14)
- *Serious bleeding* – this is usually obvious and can be brought under control (see BLEEDING, p.46)

If more than one child is injured go to the quiet one first – he may be unconscious.

4 Get help

Shout for help early to bring others to your assistance, and ask them to: • Make the area safe • Call an ambulance • Help with first aid • Move a child to safety, if necessary

Telephoning for help

When you call 911, ask for an ambulance and give the following information:
- Your telephone number
- The accident location
- The type of accident
- The number, sex, and age of the victims
- Details about their condition
- Details of any hazards such as spilled gasoline

Always let the dispatcher hang up first.

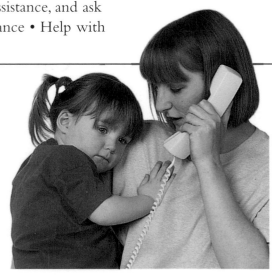

FIRE

Have an escape plan
Before an emergency happens, decide:
• *How would you get out of each room?*
• *How do you help babies and small children?*
• *Where will you meet when you've escaped?*

SKILLET FIRE *(grease fire)* • *Turn off stove* • *Cover pan with lid, wet dishtowel, or fire blanket for 30 minutes* • **DO NOT** *throw water on the flames* • *If not under control, close the door, get everyone out of the house, call the fire department.*

Escaping from a fire

1 Feel the door. If the door is cool, leave the room. If it is hot, see step 2.

REMEMBER • *Carry out babies and toddlers* • *Children over six should look after only themselves when escaping — don't ask them to do anything else.*
• *Close all doors behind you*
• *Meet outside your house*
• *NEVER go back inside* • *Phone for help from somewhere else*

2 If the door is hot, don't open it. Go to the window.

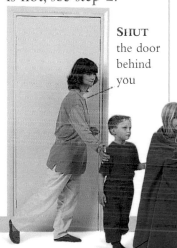

SHUT the door behind you

LEAVE quickly
DO NOT GO BACK

IF *you have to escape through the window, slide your child out, hang onto him, then ask him to drop to the ground. Slide out yourself, hang from the ledge, then drop. If you have to break the glass first, put a blanket over the frame before escaping.*

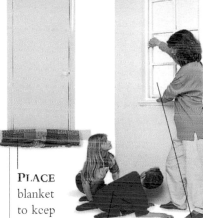

PLACE blanket to keep smoke out

KEEP children low, where air is clearest

OPEN window, call for help; hang towel to attract attention

Clothing on fire

If clothing is on fire:
Stop your child from moving since movement will fan flames.
Drop him to the floor to prevent his face and airway burning.
Wrap him in a coat or blanket to help smother the flames.
Roll him on the ground to put out the fire.

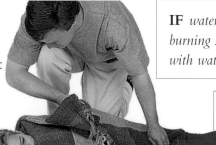

IF *water is available, lay him down, burning side uppermost, and douse him with water or a nonflammable liquid.*

DO NOT *let your child run about in a panic; rapid movement will fan the flames.*

11

ELECTRICAL INJURY

If an electrical current passes through a child's body, it may cause breathing and even the heart to stop. The current may cause burns both where it enters and leaves the body. Alternating current (AC) causes muscle spasms that can prevent a child from letting go of an electric cord.

CONTACT *with high-voltage current, found in power lines and overhead cables, is usually fatal for a child. Severe burns result and the child may be thrown some distance from the point of contact.* **NEVER** *approach the injured child unless you are told officially that the power has been cut off, or you will be in danger from "arcing," or "jumping," high-voltage electricity.*

Low-voltage current

Children are at risk of suffering an electric shock if they play with electrical sockets or wires, or if they bring an electric appliance into contact with water.

IF *the child seems unharmed, make him rest and observe his condition.* © CALL A DOCTOR

1 Break the contact by switching off the current at the circuit breaker.

2 If you cannot switch off the current, stand on dry insulating material such as telephone books or a wooden box. Use a wooden broom handle or chair to push your child's limbs away from the source.

IF *your child loses consciousness, assess his condition (see UNCONSCIOUS BABY, p.16; UNCONSCIOUS CHILD, p.22). Cool burns with cold water (see ELECTRICAL BURNS, p.62). Be prepared to resuscitate. If breathing, place him in the RECOVERY POSITION (p.24).*

DO NOT *touch your child's skin with your hands. Pull at his clothes only as a last resort.*

STAND on insulating material

PUSH the source away

3 Without touching your child, wrap a dry towel around his feet and pull him away from the source.

☎ CALL 911

WRAP a dry towel around his feet. Pull him away

12

DROWNING

Babies and young children can drown quickly if they slip into a pool or pond or are left unattended in a bath. Even 1in (2.5cm) of water is enough to cover a baby's nose and mouth if she falls forward.

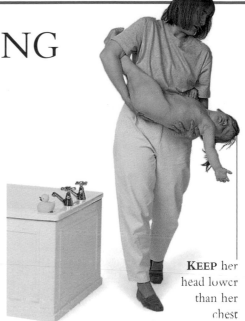

A CHILD *may get into difficulty in open water especially if it is turbulent or very cold. Rescue him quickly. Try to reach him from the shore or bank with your hand, or with a stick. Get him dry and warm up as quickly as possible (see also* HYPOTHERMIA, p. 94)*.*

1 Lift your child out of the water. Carry her with her head lower than her chest.

2 ☎ CALL 911
OR
✚ TAKE HER TO THE HOSPITAL, even if she seems to have recovered, since she may have inhaled water, causing lung damage.

KEEP her head lower than her chest

The unconscious child

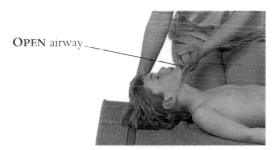

OPEN airway

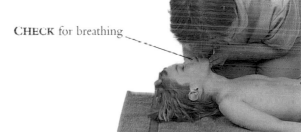

CHECK for breathing

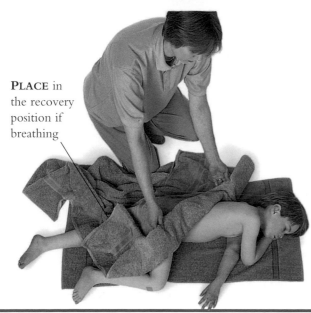

PLACE in the recovery position if breathing

Remove any wet clothing and cover him with a dry towel or blanket. Assess his condition (see UNCONSCIOUS BABY, p.16; UNCONSCIOUS CHILD, p.22). Be prepared to resuscitate. If breathing, place him in the RECOVERY POSITION, p.24).

☎ CALL 911

WATER *in the lungs and the effects of cold can increase resistance to rescue breathing so you may need to breathe more firmly and more slowly to get the chest to rise.*

13

ABC OF RESUSCITATION

A baby or child who stops breathing will become unconsious because no oxygen reaches the brain. Lack of oxygen also causes the heartbeat to slow down until it stops altogether. If your baby or child is unconscious and stops breathing, you need to open the airway and breathe into the lungs (rescue breathing). If the circulation has stopped, you need to help blood get to the brain by doing chest compressions. This combination of rescue breathing and chest compressions is known as cardiopulmonary resuscitation (CPR).

FOR *a step-by-step guide to* RESUSCITATING A BABY, *see p.16.* **FOR** *a step-by-step guide to* RESUSCITATING A CHILD, *see p.22.*

ASSESS your baby and act on your findings

ASSESS your child and act on your findings

TAP her shoulder

14

A is for airway

You need to open the airway. If the infant or child is unresponsive, and if she has not suffered a neck or head injury, tilt the head back and lift the chin. This will bring the tongue away from the back of the throat and open the airway. Look in the mouth and remove any obvious obstructions.

For a baby

For a child

Blocked airway – head not tilted

TONGUE fallen back

BLOCKED airway

Unblocked airway – head tilted and chin lifted

TONGUE forward

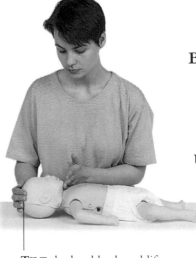

UNBLOCKED airway

TILT the head back and lift the chin to clear the airway

TILT the head back and lift the chin to clear the airway

B is for breathing

For a baby

If your child is not breathing after the airway is open, take a deep breath and blow steadily into the lungs to get oxygen into the child's blood.

For a child

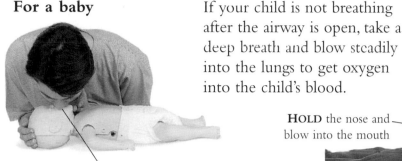

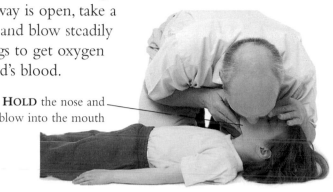

HOLD the nose and blow into the mouth

BREATHE gently into the mouth and nose until the chest rises

C is for circulation

For a baby

If there are no signs of circulation (normal breathing, coughing, or movement), giving chest compressions will drive blood through the heart and around the body. This is always combined with rescue breathing. The combination of techniques is known as cardiopulmonary resuscitation (CPR).

For a child

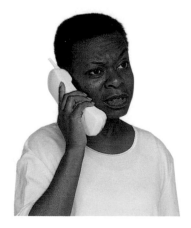

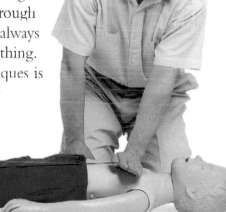

CHEST COMPRESSIONS are given with two fingers

CHEST COMPRESSIONS are given with one hand only

15

When to call 911

If there is somebody else present, always ask him or her to call 911 as soon as you realize that your child is not breathing.

If you are alone, give rescue breaths (see RESCUE BREATHING: BABY, p.18; RESCUE BREATHING:CHILD, p.26) or cardiopulmonary rescuscitation (see CPR: BABY, p.20; CPR: CHILD, p.28), as appropriate, for about one minute before pausing to call 911.

UNCONSCIOUS BABY

Assess your baby's condition

1 Check for response

- Call his name
- Tap or flick the sole of his foot

NEVER shake a baby

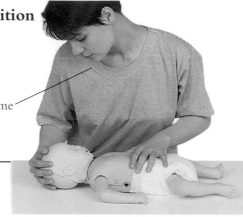

CALL his name

2 Shout for help

3 Open the airway

- Tilt your baby's head back gently
- Remove any obvious obstructions from the mouth or nose
- Use your fingertips to lift the chin

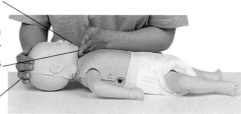

LOOK in mouth

LIFT chin with your fingertips

TILT head back gently

4 Check for breathing

- Listen for sounds of breathing
- Feel for breath on your cheek
- Look along the chest for movement
- Check for no more than ten seconds
- If breathing, go straight to step 6 (opposite)

IF NOT *breathing, give two effective rescue breaths (see p.18), then proceed to step 5 (below).*

PUT your mouth over baby's mouth and nose

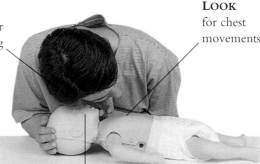

LISTEN for breathing

LOOK for chest movements

FEEL for breath on your cheek

5 Check for signs of circulation

- Look for breathing, coughing, and movement for no more than ten seconds

6 Act on your findings

Baby unconscious, breathing and signs of circulation present

1 Treat any life-threatening injuries such as severe bleeding (p.46).

2 Cradle your baby in your arms with his head tilted down (the recovery position).

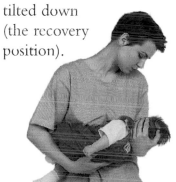

3 ☎ CALL 911
Ask a helper to do this. If you have no helper, take your baby with you to the telephone.

4 Keep your baby in your arms until help arrives. Keep checking his breathing.

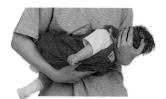

Not breathing but signs of circulation present

1 Continue to give rescue breaths (mouth to-mouth-and-nose) for about one minute (see next page).

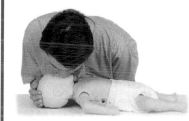

2 ☎ CALL 911
Take your baby with you to the telephone, if necessary.

3 Continue giving rescue breaths until help arrives.

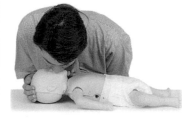

4 Check for signs of circulation every minute.

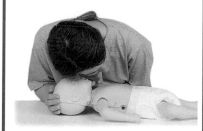

Not breathing, no signs of circulation

1 Give cardiopulmonary resuscitation (CPR) – five chest compressions followed by one rescue breath (mouth-to-mouth-and-nose) – at a rate of at least 100 per minute, for one minute (see p.20).

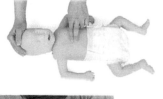

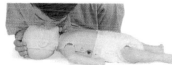

2 ☎ CALL 911
Take your baby with you to the telephone, if necessary.

3 Continue giving cardiopulmonary resuscitation (CPR) until help arrives.

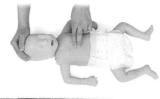

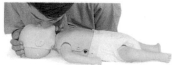

RESCUE BREATHING: BABY

To be used for an unconscious baby who is not breathing, before you check for signs of circulation (see p.16).

RESUSCITATION SUMMARY

UNCONSCIOUS BABY

AIRWAY OPEN

NO BREATHING

GIVE 2 EFFECTIVE **RESCUE BREATHS**

SIGNS OF CIRCULATION PRESENT

GIVE **RESCUE BREATHS** FOR 1 MINUTE

☎ CALL 911

CONTINUE GIVING **RESCUE BREATHS** UNTIL HELP ARRIVES

18

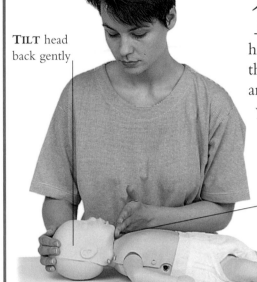

TILT head back gently

LIFT point of chin with one finger

1 Make sure your baby is on his back on a firm surface. Tilt his head back gently and check that his airway is open. Pick out any obvious obstruction with your fingertips, but do not do a finger sweep. Lift his chin using one finger.

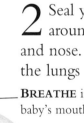

BREATHE into the baby's mouth and nose

LET the chest rise

2 Seal your lips tightly around your baby's mouth and nose. Breathe gently into the lungs until the chest rises.

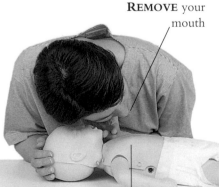

REMOVE your mouth

WATCH the chest fall back

3 Remove your mouth and let the chest fall back. A breath is effective if the chest rises and falls.

IF *your baby's chest does not rise, check his mouth again and adjust the position of his head.*

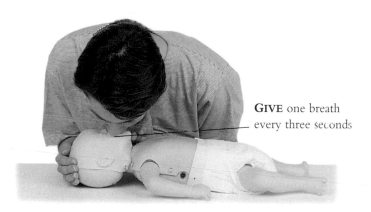

GIVE one breath
every three seconds

4 Repeat rescue breaths up
to five times if necessary, to
achieve two effective breaths.

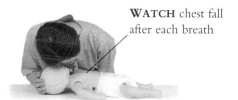

WATCH chest fall
after each breath

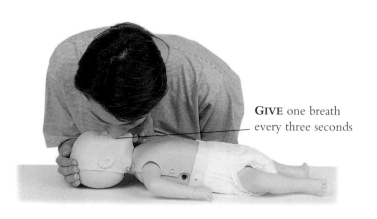

LOOK for breathing,
coughing, or movement

5 Stop and check for signs of
circulation (see p.16). If these
are absent, start cardiopulmonary
resuscitation (CPR, see next
page). Otherwise, continue
to give rescue breaths for one
minute, aiming for one complete
breath every three seconds
(about 20 breaths per minute).

6 ☎ CALL 911
Take your baby with you to
the telephone, if necessary.

7 Continue to give rescue
breaths until help arrives.
Check for signs of circulation
every minute. If absent, start
CPR (see next page).

GIVE one breath
every three seconds

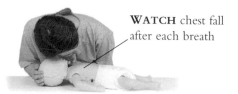

WATCH chest fall
after each breath

19

CPR ^(CARDIOPULMONARY RESUSCITATION) : BABY

To be used when an unconscious baby is not breathing and has no signs of circulation (see p.16). Give CPR for a full minute before you call an ambulance.

RESUSCITATION SUMMARY

UNCONSCIOUS BABY

AIRWAY OPEN

NO BREATHING

GIVE 2 EFFECTIVE RESCUE BREATHS (see p.18)

NO SIGNS OF CIRCULATION

CPR – 5 CHEST COMPRESSIONS, 1 RESCUE BREATH – REPEATED FOR 1 MINUTE

☎ CALL 911

CONTINUE **CPR** UNTIL HELP ARRIVES

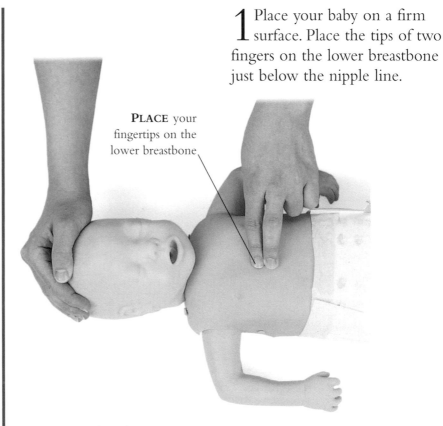

1 Place your baby on a firm surface. Place the tips of two fingers on the lower breastbone just below the nipple line.

PLACE your fingertips on the lower breastbone

PRESS down by one-third to one-half of the depth of the chest

2 Press down sharply by one-third to one-half of the depth of the chest. Do this five times at a rate of at least 100 compressions per minute.

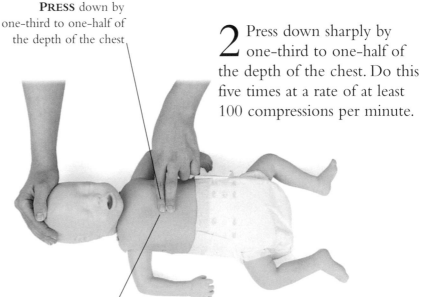

GIVE 5 compressions

20

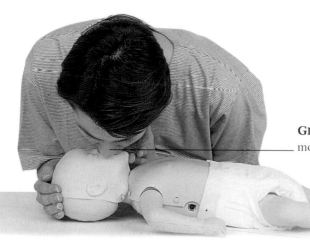

3 Give one rescue breath (see p.18).

GIVE one breath of mouth-to-mouth-and-nose

Repeat steps 2 and 3 for about a minute

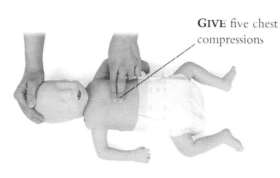

GIVE five chest compressions

4 Continue the cycle of five chest compressions to one rescue breath for about one minute.

FOLLOW with one breath

Repeat CPR cycles until help arrives

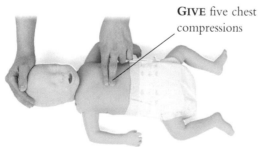

GIVE five chest compressions

5 ☎ CALL 911
If you have no helper, take your baby with you to the telephone.

6 Continue giving CPR – five chest compressions followed by one rescue breath – until the ambulance arrives.

DO NOT *stop to make circulation checks unless your baby makes a movement or takes a spontaneous breath. If breathing and circulation return, cradle your baby in your arms with his head tilted down (see p.17) and monitor him carefully until the ambulance arrives.*

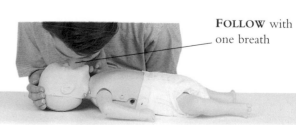

FOLLOW with one breath

21

UNCONSCIOUS CHILD

Assess your child's condition

1 Check for response
- Call her name
- Tap her shoulder gently

IF *you suspect BACK AND NECK INJURIES, see pp. 74–75.*

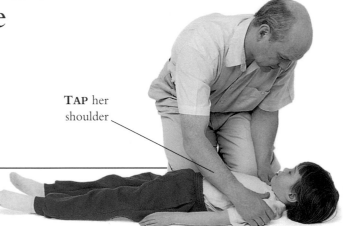

TAP her shoulder

2 Shout for help

3 Open the airway
- Place one hand on the forehead and gently tilt the head back
- Remove any obvious obstruction from the mouth.
- Use two fingers to lift the chin

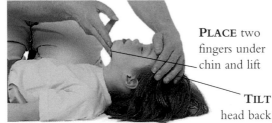

PLACE two fingers under chin and lift

TILT head back

4 Check for breathing
- Listen for sounds of breathing
- Feel for breath on your cheek
- Look along the chest for movement
- Check for no more than ten seconds
- If breathing, go straight to step 6 (opposite)

IF NOT *breathing, give two effective rescue breaths (see p.26), then proceed to step 5 (below).*

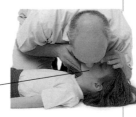

PUT your mouth over child's mouth and breathe

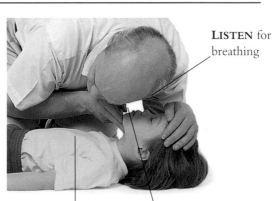

LISTEN for breathing

LOOK for chest movements

FEEL for breath on your cheek

5 Check for signs of circulation
- Look for breathing, coughing, and movement for no more than ten seconds

22

6 Act on your findings

Child unconscious, breathing and signs of circulation present

1 Treat any life-threatening injuries such as severe bleeding (see p.46).

2 Place her in the recovery position (see pp.24–25).

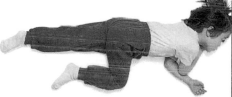

3 ☎ CALL 911

4 Keep checking her breathing until help arrives and be prepared to resuscitate.

Not breathing but signs of circulation present

1 Continue to give rescue breaths (mouth-to-mouth) for about one minute (see p.26).

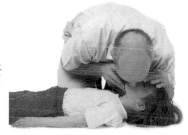

2 ☎ CALL 911

3 Continue to give rescue breaths until help arrives.

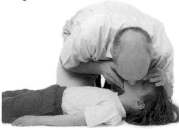

4 Check for signs of circulation every minute (after every 20 breaths).

Not breathing, no signs of circulation

1 Give cardiopulmonary resuscitation (CPR) – five chest compressions followed by one rescue breath (mouth-to-mouth) – for one minute (see p.28).

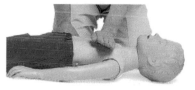

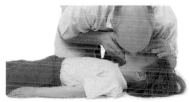

2 ☎ CALL 911

3 Continue giving cardiopulmonary resuscitation (CPR) until help arrives.

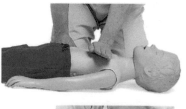

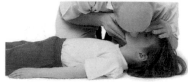

23

RECOVERY POSITION

Put your child in this position if she is unconscious, breathing, and has signs of circulation (see p.22) to keep her from choking on her tongue or vomit.

BE *very careful if you think there is a broken bone. Move her so the injured side is uppermost. See BONE, JOINT, AND MUSCLE INJURIES, pp.76–84.*

IF *you suspect BACK AND NECK INJURIES, see pp.74–75.*

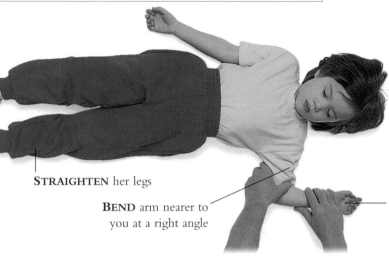

1 Kneel beside your child. Remove glasses and any bulky objects from her pockets. If necessary, straighten her legs. Bend the arm nearest you so that it makes a right angle and lay it on the ground, with the palm of the hand upward.

STRAIGHTEN her legs

BEND arm nearer to you at a right angle

PLACE back of her hand on the ground

2 Bring her other arm across her chest. Hold the back of her hand against her opposite cheek.

MOVE farther arm across her chest and bend it

PLACE back of her hand against her cheek

PLACE her foot flat on ground

CLASP under thigh of outside leg and bend at knee

3 Use your free hand to clasp gently under the thigh that is farther from you. Carefully pull the knee up to bend the leg, leaving the foot flat on the ground.

KEEP this leg straight

SUPPORT her hand against her cheek

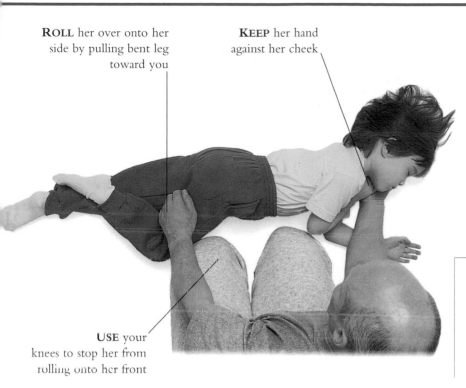

ROLL her over onto her side by pulling bent leg toward you

KEEP her hand against her cheek

USE your knees to stop her from rolling onto her front

4 Keep your child's hand against her cheek to support her head. At the same time, pull on the thigh of the bent leg to roll your child toward you and onto her side.

IF *your child is already lying on her side or is on her front, you will need to adapt these steps when placing her in the recovery position.*

CHECK *your child's breathing and circulation frequently while you are waiting for help to arrive.*

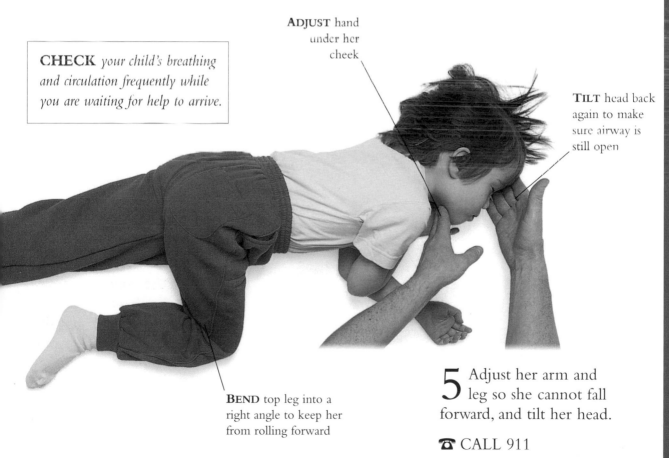

ADJUST hand under her cheek

TILT head back again to make sure airway is still open

BEND top leg into a right angle to keep her from rolling forward

5 Adjust her arm and leg so she cannot fall forward, and tilt her head.

☎ CALL 911

RESCUE BREATHING: CHILD

To be used for an unconscious child who is not breathing, before you check for signs of circulation (see p.22).

**RESUSCITATION
SUMMARY**

UNCONSCIOUS CHILD

AIRWAY OPEN

NO BREATHING

GIVE 2 EFFECTIVE
RESCUE BREATHS

SIGNS OF
CIRCULATION
PRESENT

GIVE
RESCUE BREATHS
FOR 1 MINUTE

☎ CALL 911

CONTINUE GIVING
RESCUE BREATHS
UNTIL HELP
ARRIVES

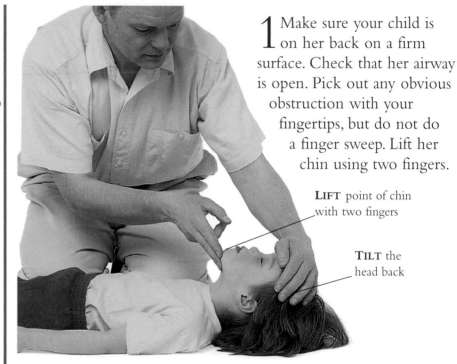

1 Make sure your child is on her back on a firm surface. Check that her airway is open. Pick out any obvious obstruction with your fingertips, but do not do a finger sweep. Lift her chin using two fingers.

LIFT point of chin with two fingers

TILT the head back

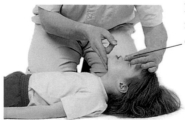

PINCH nostrils closed

2 Pinch her nostrils closed. Seal your lips round her open mouth. Breathe into the lungs until you see the chest rise.

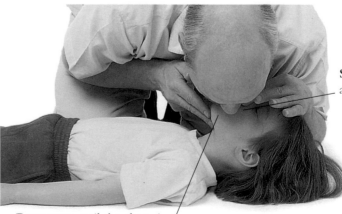

SEAL your lips around her mouth

BREATHE until the chest rises

26

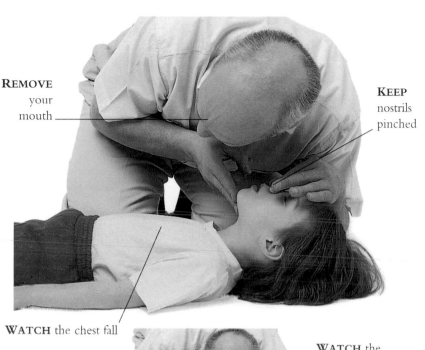

REMOVE
your
mouth

KEEP
nostrils
pinched

WATCH the chest fall

3 Remove your mouth and let the chest fall. Keep the nostrils pinched. A breath is effective if the chest rises and falls.

> **IF** *your child's chest does not rise, check her mouth again and adjust the position of her head.*

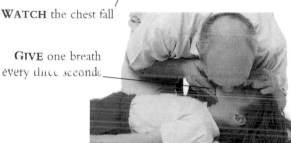

GIVE one breath
every three seconds

WATCH the
chest fall

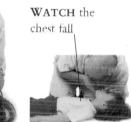

4 Repeat rescue breaths up to five times if necessary, to achieve two effective breaths.

27

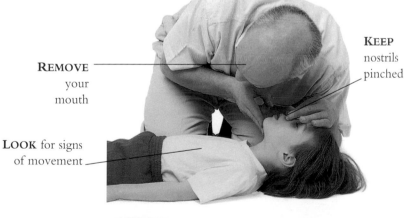

REMOVE
your
mouth

LOOK for signs
of movement

KEEP
nostrils
pinched

5 Stop and check for signs of circulation (see p.22). If these are absent, start CPR (cardiopulmonary resuscitation, see next page). Otherwise, continue to give rescue breaths for one minute, aiming for one complete breath every three seconds (about 20 breaths per minute).

6 ☎ CALL 911

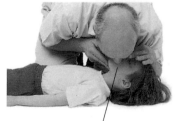

GIVE one breath
every three seconds

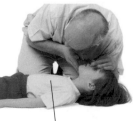

WATCH the chest
fall after each breath

7 Continue to give rescue breaths until help arrives. Check for signs of circulation every minute. If absent, start CPR (see next page).

CPR (CARDIOPULMONARY RESUSCITATION) : CHILD

To be used when an unconscious child is not breathing and has no signs of circulation (see p.22). Give CPR for a full minute before you call an ambulance.

RESUSCITATION SUMMARY

UNCONSCIOUS CHILD

⬇

AIRWAY OPEN

⬇

NO BREATHING

⬇

GIVE 2 EFFECTIVE RESCUE BREATHS
(see p.26)

⬇

NO SIGNS OF CIRCULATION

⬇

CPR – 5 CHEST COMPRESSIONS, 1 RESCUE BREATH – REPEATED FOR 1 MINUTE

⬇

☎ CALL 911

⬇

CONTINUE **CPR** UNTIL HELP ARRIVES

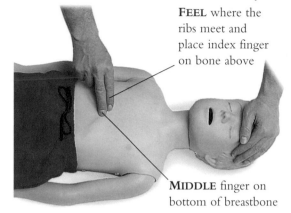

FEEL where the ribs meet and place index finger on bone above

MIDDLE finger on bottom of breastbone

1 Place your child on her back on a firm surface. Find the point on the chest where the ribs meet (breastbone). Put your middle finger on the bottom of the breastbone, your index finger on the bone above.

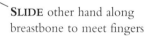

SLIDE other hand along breastbone to meet fingers

2 Slide the heel of your other hand down the breastbone to meet your fingers.

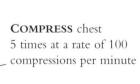

PRESS down by one-third to one-half of the depth of the chest

3 Using the heel of one hand only, press down sharply at this point by one-third to one-half of the depth of the chest. Do this five times at a rate of 100 compressions per minute.

COMPRESS chest 5 times at a rate of 100 compressions per minute

28

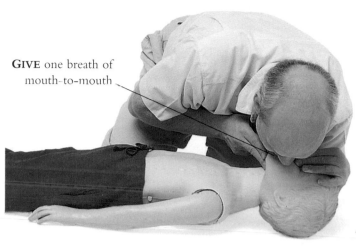

GIVE one breath of mouth-to-mouth

4 Give one rescue breath (see p.26).

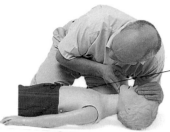

WATCH chest fall

Repeat steps 3 and 4 for about a minute

5 Continue the CPR cycle of five chest compressions to one rescue breath for about one minute.

GIVE five chest compressions

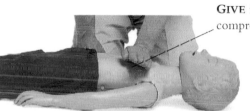

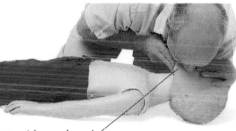

FOLLOW with one breath

Repeat CPR cycles until help arrives

GIVE five chest compressions

6 ☎ CALL 911

FOLLOW with one breath

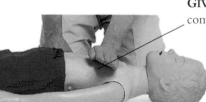

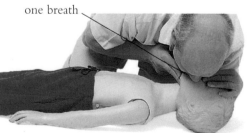

DO NOT *stop to make circulation checks unless your child makes a movement or takes a spontaneous breath. If breathing and circulation return, place your child in the RECOVERY POSITION (see p.24) and monitor her carefully until the ambulance arrives.*

7 Continue giving CPR – five chest compressions followed by one rescue breath – until the ambulance arrives.

29

SHOCK

Recognizing shock This develops from the early signs of • *Pale, cold, and sweaty skin, tinged with gray* • *Rapid pulse becoming weaker* • *Shallow, fast breathing,* to the later signs of • *Restlessness, yawning, and sighing* • *Thirst* • *Loss of consciousness*

THE *most likely cause of shock in a child is serious BLEEDING, see p.46, or a SEVERE BURN OR SCALD, see p.60. These injuries must be treated without delay.*

DO NOT *give your child anything to drink or eat. If he is thirsty, moisten his lips with water.*

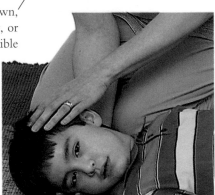

MOVE your child as little as possible

LAY him down, on blanket, coat, or rug, if possible

KEEP his head flat on floor

1 Lay your child down flat. Keep his head low since this improves the blood supply to the brain. Reassure him. Treat any injury.

☎ CALL 911

2 Carefully raise your child's legs 8–12 inches and support them with pillows, or on a pile of books padded with a cushion.

KEEP his head lower than his chest

REASSURE him

RAISE his legs high above heart level

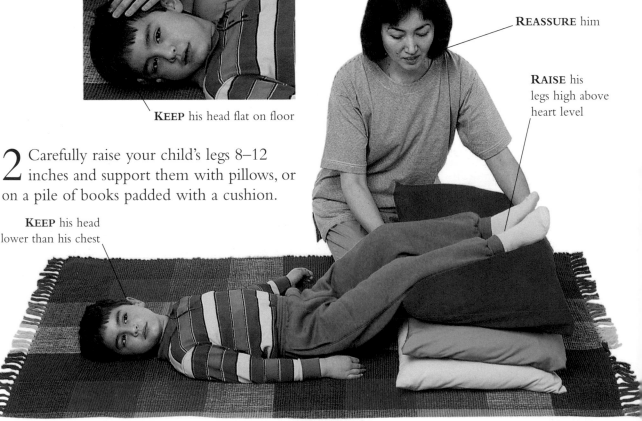

30

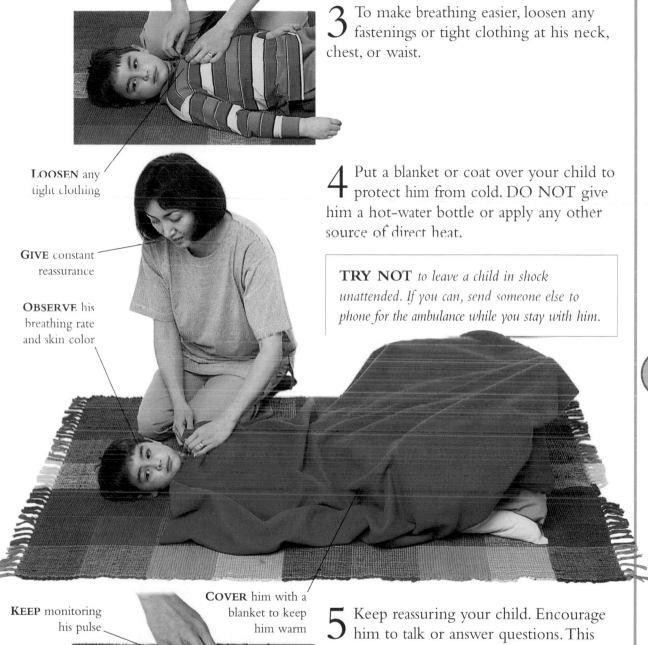

3 To make breathing easier, loosen any fastenings or tight clothing at his neck, chest, or waist.

LOOSEN any tight clothing

GIVE constant reassurance

OBSERVE his breathing rate and skin color

4 Put a blanket or coat over your child to protect him from cold. DO NOT give him a hot-water bottle or apply any other source of direct heat.

TRY NOT *to leave a child in shock unattended. If you can, send someone else to phone for the ambulance while you stay with him.*

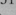

KEEP monitoring his pulse

COVER him with a blanket to keep him warm

5 Keep reassuring your child. Encourage him to talk or answer questions. This will help you assess his condition. Note any changes and tell the ambulance personnel.

IF *he loses consciousness, assess his condition (see UNCONSCIOUS BABY, p.16; UNCONSCIOUS CHILD, p.22). Be prepared to resuscitate. If breathing, place him in the RECOVERY POSITION.*

FEBRILE SEIZURES

Young children may develop these seizures when they have an infection and a high temperature.

Recognizing a seizure • *She may be flushed and sweating with a very hot forehead* • *Her eyes may roll upward, or be fixed or squinting* • *Her face may look blue if she is holding her breath* • *She may stiffen and arch her back* • *Her fists may clench*

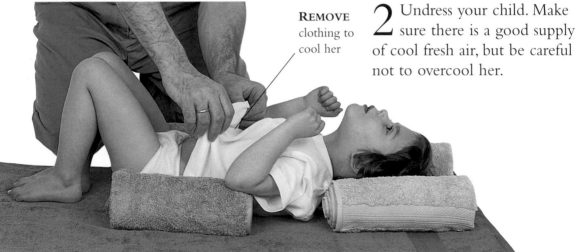

PROTECT her with padding

1 Place soft padding, such as towels or pillows, around your child so that even violent movement will not lead to injury.

REMOVE clothing to cool her

2 Undress your child. Make sure there is a good supply of cool fresh air, but be careful not to overcool her.

3 When your child is cooled, seizures will stop. Place her in the RECOVERY POSITION (see p.24). Cover her with a light blanket or sheet and reassure her. If her temperature rises, cool her again.

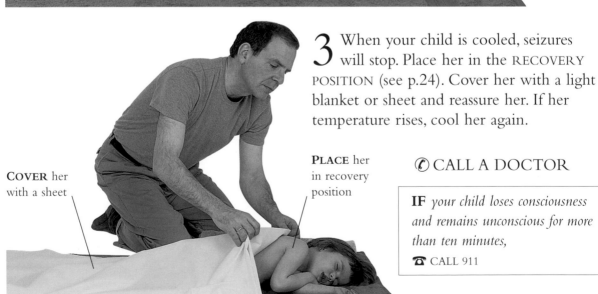

COVER her with a sheet

PLACE her in recovery position

✆ CALL A DOCTOR

IF *your child loses consciousness and remains unconscious for more than ten minutes,*
☎ CALL 911

EPILEPTIC SEIZURES

Recognizing major epilepsy A seizure may progress through the following stages:
• *Sudden loss of unconsciousness, sometimes with a cry* • *Rigidity and arching of back* • *Breathing may stop* • *Jerking movements* • *Froth or bubbles around the mouth, may be blood-stained* • *Bladder or bowel control lost* • *Conscious within a few minutes* • *Dazed feeling* • *Deep sleep may follow*

Children with a history of epilepsy may have a card or bracelet alerting you to this. A child may have a minor seizure before a major one. This can be recognized by a momentary "switching off," some facial twitching, or distracted movements such as lip-smacking. If this happens, reassure the child and arrange to see your doctor.

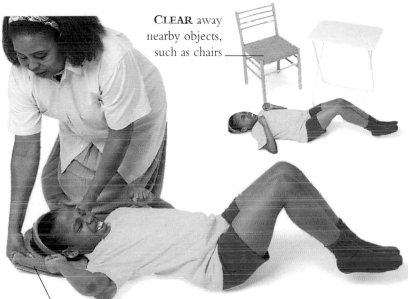

CLEAR away nearby objects, such as chairs

PROTECT her head with soft padding

1 If your child starts to fall, help her to the floor. Clear away objects that she may knock against. Place padding under or around her head. Do not hold her down or try to move her. Don't put anything in her mouth or give her anything to eat or drink.

Once the seizure has stopped

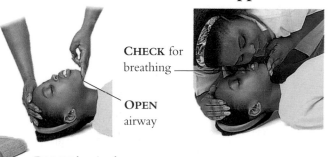

CHECK for breathing

OPEN airway

PLACE her in the recovery position if breathing

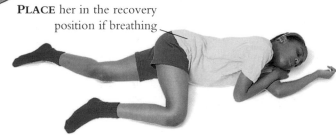

2 When her seizure is over, your child may be unconscious. Remove any padding and assess her (see p. 22). If breathing, place her in the RECOVERY POSITION (see p.24). Stay with her until she is recovered. She may feel dazed and behave strangely, or sleep deeply.

✆ CALL A DOCTOR

> **IF** *your child has never had a seizure before, if she has repeated seizures, or if she remains unconscious for more than ten minutes,*
> ☎ CALL 911

33

DIABETIC EMERGENCY

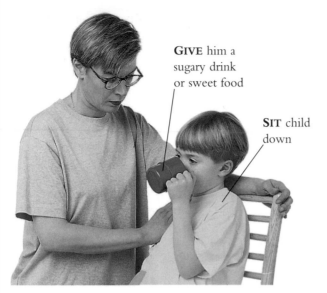

GIVE him a sugary drink or sweet food

SIT child down

Recognizing low blood sugar

• Weakness or hunger • Confused or aggressive behavior • Sweating • Very pale face • Strong, bounding pulse • Shallow breathing

> *A child who is diabetic is likely to be on insulin. Even if he seems recovered, a doctor should be asked to check the insulin dosage.*

If he improves rapidly after a sweet drink or food, give him some more and let him rest. If he does not improve,
☎ CALL 911

An unconscious child

34

OPEN airway

CHECK for breathing

1 Open the airway and check that breathing is present.

> **IF** *your child is not breathing, be prepared to resuscitate (see* UNCONSCIOUS BABY, *p.16;* UNCONSCIOUS CHILD, *p.22).*

2 If she is breathing, place her in the RECOVERY POSITION (see p.24).

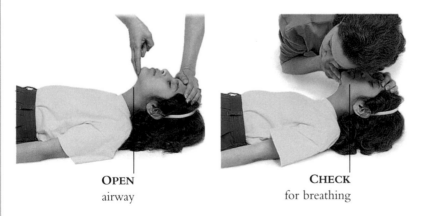

PLACE her in the recovery position if breathing

☎ CALL 911

FAINT

RAISE her legs to improve blood flow to her brain

Recognizing a faint • *Child feels weak, giddy, and nauseous* • *Very pale face* • *Brief loss of consciousness* • *Slow pulse*

1 Lay your child down and raise her legs above the level of her heart, supporting them on a pile of cushions, pillows, or folded blankets about 8–12 inches high.

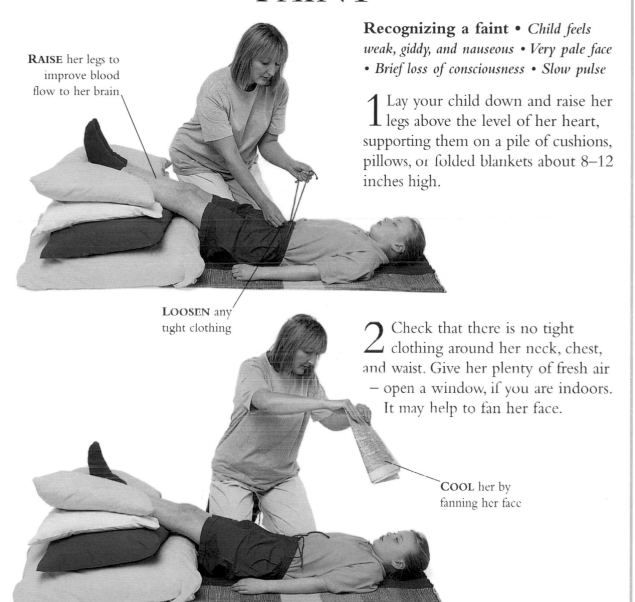

LOOSEN any tight clothing

2 Check that there is no tight clothing around her neck, chest, and waist. Give her plenty of fresh air – open a window, if you are indoors. It may help to fan her face.

COOL her by fanning her face

35

PLACE her in the recovery position if she is slow to regain consciousness

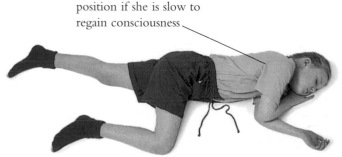

3 If your child does not regain consciousness, assess her condition (see UNCONSCIOUS BABY, p.16; UNCONSCIOUS CHILD, p.22). Be prepared to resuscitate. If breathing, place her in the RECOVERY POSITION.

☎ CALL 911

CHOKING: CONSCIOUS BABY

SUMMARY

GIVE 5
BACK BLOWS

CHECK MOUTH

GIVE 5 CHEST
THRUSTS

CHECK MOUTH

Repeat cycle of 5 back blows,
mouth check, 5 chest thrusts,
mouth check, three times

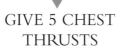 CALL 911

Repeat cycle until
help arrives or the
obstruction clears

DO NOT *shake a baby*

Recognizing a choking baby • *Breathing is obstructed* • *Trying to cry but making strange noises, or no sound* • *Face may turn blue*

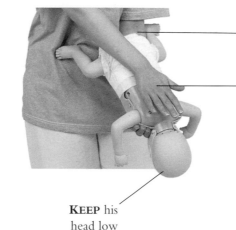

LAY him along
your forearm

GIVE five back
blows

KEEP his
head low

1 Lay your baby face
down with his head
low along your forearm.
Support his head and
shoulders on your hand.
Give five back blows to
the upper part of his back.

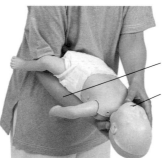

TURN HIM
onto his back
along your
other arm

LOOK IN
his mouth
and remove
any object
you can see

2 Turn him face up
along your other
arm. Look inside his
mouth and remove any
obvious obstruction
with one finger. Do not
feel blindly down your
baby's throat.

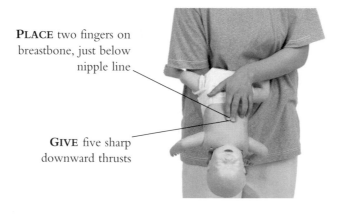

PLACE two fingers on
breastbone, just below
nipple line

GIVE five sharp
downward thrusts

3 If back blows fail,
place two fingers on
the lower half of your
baby's breastbone and
give five sharp downward
thrusts at a rate of one
every second. These act
as artificial coughs.
Check the mouth again.

4 If the blockage hasn't cleared, repeat steps 1–3
three times. Take your baby with you and
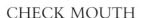 CALL 911

CHOKING: UNCONSCIOUS BABY

If your baby becomes unconscious

Open the airway and check breathing (see p.16). If breathing, carefully remove any visible obstruction from the mouth. Cradle your baby in your arms with his head tilted down (see p.17).
☎ CALL 911
Keep your baby in your arms and continue to check his breathing until help arrives.

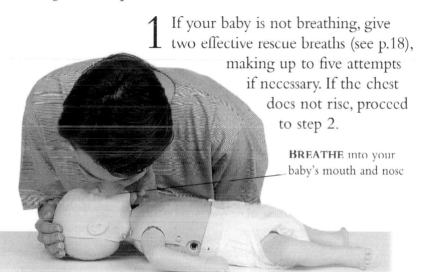

1 If your baby is not breathing, give two effective rescue breaths (see p.18), making up to five attempts if necessary. If the chest does not rise, proceed to step 2.

BREATHE into your baby's mouth and nose

SUMMARY

GIVE 2 RESCUE BREATHS

CHEST DOES NOT RISE

CPR – 5 CHEST COMPRESSIONS, 1 RESCUE BREATH REPEATED FOR 1 MINUTE

☎ CALL 911

Continue CPR until help arrives or the baby resumes breathing

37

2 Give five chest compressions (see CPR, p.20) in an attempt to dislodge the obstruction. Then check the mouth and give one rescue breath. Repeat steps 1 and 2 for one minute.

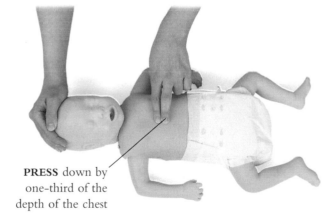

PRESS down by one-third of the depth of the chest

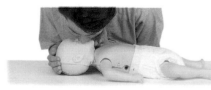

☎ CALL 911

Repeat CPR cycle until help arrives

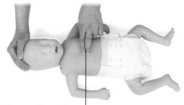

GIVE five chest compressions

FOLLOW with one breath

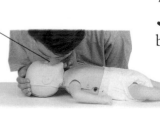

3 Continue CPR until help arrives or your baby resumes breathing.

CHOKING: CONSCIOUS CHILD

SUMMARY

ENCOURAGE CHILD TO COUGH

GIVE 5 ABDOMINAL THRUSTS

CHECK MOUTH

Repeat cycle of mouth check, 5 abdominal thrusts, mouth check, three times

☎ CALL 911

Continue cycle until help arrives or the blockage is expelled

Recognizing a choking child • *Sudden clutching at the throat* • *Child unable to speak or breathe* • *Face may go blue*

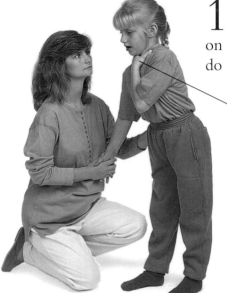

1 Your child may be able to cough up the obsruction on her own. Encourage her to do this, but do not waste time.

GET her to cough up obstruction if she can

2 Check her mouth. Put your finger on the tongue for a clear view. Remove any object you can see.

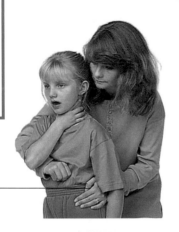

3 Stand or kneel behind her, and wrap your arms around her waist. Make a fist with one hand. Place the thumb side of your fist against the middle of her abdomen, just above her navel.

STAND behind her and wrap your arms around her waist

4 Give up to five upward and inward thrusts. Check the mouth.

PRESS into her abdomen with quick upward thrusts

5 If the abdominal thrusts fail, repeat steps 2–3 three times. If this is unsuccessful, ☎ CALL 911

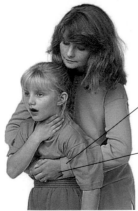

MAKE a fist and grasp it with your other hand

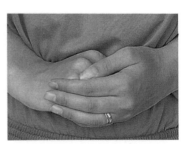

PRESS the thumb side of your fist just above her navel. Grasp fist with the other hand.

Continue the above cycle until help arrives or the obstruction is cleared.

38

CHOKING: UNCONSCIOUS CHILD

If your child becomes unconscious

Open the airway and check breathing (see p.22). If breathing, carefully remove any visible obstruction from the mouth. Place your child in the recovery position (see p.24).

☎ CALL 911

Keep checking his breathing until help arrives.

SUMMARY

GIVE 2 RESCUE BREATHS

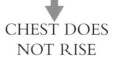

CHEST DOES NOT RISE

CPR 5 CHEST COMPRESSIONS, 1 RESCUE BREATH FOR 1 MINUTE

☎ CALL 911

Continue CPR until help arrives or the child resumes breathing

1 If your child is not breathing, give two effective rescue breaths (see p.26), making up to five attempts if necessary. If the chest does not rise, proceed to step 2.

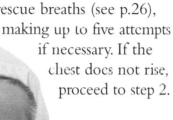

GIVE two rescue breaths

2 Give five chest compressions (see CPR, p.28) in an attempt to dislodge the obstruction. Then check the mouth and give one rescue breath. Repeat steps 1 and 2 for one minute.

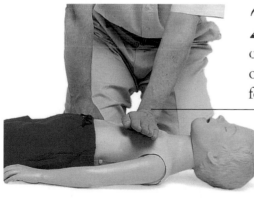

COMPRESS chest five times at a rate of 100 compressions per minute

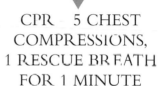

☎ CALL 911

GIVE five chest compressions

Repeat CPR cycle until help arrives

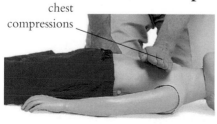

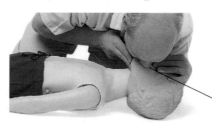

3 Continue CPR until help arrives or your child resumes breathing.

FOLLOW with one rescue breath

BREATH HOLDING

Recognizing breath holding Only children under four years of age are likely to do this. • *Your child cries, breathes in but does not breathe out* • *He may go blue in the face and stiff* • *He may become unconscious momentarily*

Breath holding is the result of rage and frustration. Try to stay calm. Do not shake him or make a fuss; walk away. He will usually start breathing again spontaneously. If he loses consciousness, see UNCONSCIOUS BABY, p.16; UNCONSCIOUS CHILD, p.22.

☎ CALL 911

HICCUPS

TELL your child to sit quietly

URGE her to hold her breath for as long as possible

OR

An older child may be able to halt the attack by drinking from the wrong side of a cup.
IF *the hiccups go on for longer than a few hours,* Ⓒ CALL A DOCTOR, *because a long attack can be worrying, tiring, and painful.*

ASK her to hold a paper bag over her mouth and nose

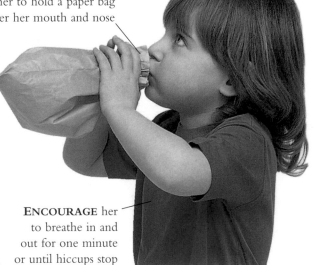

Tell your child to sit still and to hold her breath for as long as she can. Repeat this until the hiccups have gone.
OR
Hold a paper bag over her face so that she is rebreathing her own expired air. Get her to breathe in and out for about one minute.

ENCOURAGE her to breathe in and out for one minute or until hiccups stop

40

SUFFOCATION

This occurs when there is an obstruction over the mouth or nose, a weight on the child's chest or abdomen preventing normal breathing, or because the child is breathing in smoke- or fume-filled air.

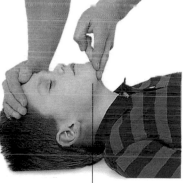

REMOVE
obstruction

1 Remove the obstruction as quickly as possible. This may restore breathing.

CHECK for breathing

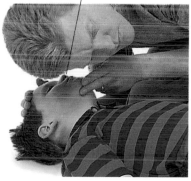

2 Open the airway. Place one hand on your child's forehead and gently tilt his head back. Remove any obvious obstruction from his mouth and lift his chin using two fingers. Look and listen for breathing for up to ten seconds.

OPEN airway

IF *your child is not breathing, see UNCONSCIOUS BABY, p.16; UNCONSCIOUS CHILD, p.22. Be prepared to resuscitate.*

3 If he is breathing, place him in the RECOVERY POSITION (see p.24).

PLACE him in the recovery position if breathing

☎ CALL 911
Continue to check your child's breathing and signs of circulation.

41

STRANGULATION

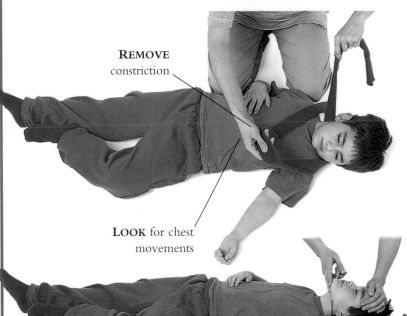

REMOVE constriction

LOOK for chest movements

1 Remove the constriction from around your child's neck without delay. Use scissors or a knife if necessary.

> **IF** *your child is hanging, support his body while you remove the rope or cord.*

2 Open the airway. Place one hand on his forehead and gently tilt his head back. Remove any obvious obstruction from his mouth and lift his chin using two fingers.

OPEN airway

42

LOOK for chest movements

KEEP the head tilted back

CHECK for breathing

3 Look and listen for breathing for up to ten seconds.

> **IF** *your child is not breathing, see UNCONSCIOUS BABY, p.16; UNCONSCIOUS CHILD, p.22. Be prepared to resuscitate.*

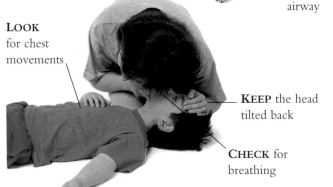

4 If he is breathing, place him in the RECOVERY POSITION (see p.24).

☎ CALL 911

Keep monitoring his breathing and signs of circulation.

> **IF** *you suspect BACK OR NECK INJURIES, see pp.74–75.*

PLACE him in the recovery position if breathing

SMOKE INHALATION

Smoke, gas, and fume inhalation requires urgent medical attention.

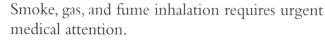 CALL 911

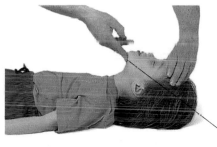

LOOK for chest movements

MOVE your child into fresh air

1 Carry your child away from the area of danger. Ensure that you do not put yourself at risk.

> **IF** *your child has any burns, see p.60.*

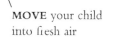

OPEN airway

2 Open the airway. Place one hand on her forehead and gently tilt her head back. Remove any obvious obstruction from her mouth and lift her chin using two fingers.

3 Check for breathing. Feel for breath on your face and look for chest movements for up to ten seconds.

CHECK for breathing

> **IF** *your child is not breathing, see* UNCONSCIOUS BABY, *p.16;* UNCONSCIOUS CHILD, *p.22. Be prepared to resuscitate.*

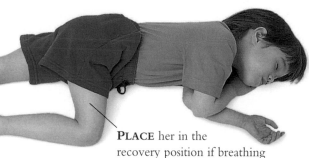

PLACE her in the recovery position if breathing

4 If your child is breathing, place her in the RECOVERY POSITION (see p.24) while you wait for help to arrive. Continue to monitor her breathing and signs of circulation.

43

CROUP

Recognizing croup This usually occurs at night. It may be alarming, but usually passes quickly. • *Difficulty breathing, particularly inhaling* • *Short, barking cough* • *Crowing or whistling noise* • *Hoarse voice.* In a severe attack • *Evidence that the child is using muscles around the nose, neck, and upper arms in his attempts to breathe* • *Blue-tinged skin*

SIT him up, supporting his back and head

BRING him into a steamy atmosphere to ease his breathing

KEEP your child away from hot running water

IF *the attack is severe and affects an older child, there is a slight risk that he is suffering a rare crouplike condition called epiglottitis. Suspect epiglottitis if your child has a high temperature and is sitting bolt upright, obviously in distress.*

☎ CALL 911

1 Help your child sit up in bed. Prop him up with pillows at his back and head and reassure him.

2 Create a steamy atmosphere; run hot water in the bathtub or shower. Try to get your child to relax enough to breathe in the steam.

OR

3 Take your child outside to breathe in cold air for about 20 minutes.

IF *the attack is severe or prolonged, lasting more than 20 minutes after Step 2 or 3,*

☎ CALL 911

Try to stay calm; if you panic this may alarm your child and worsen the attack.

44

ASTHMA

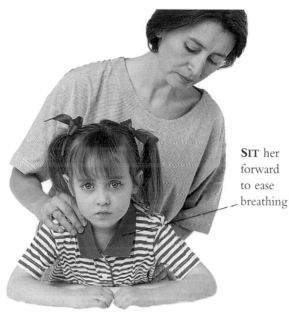

SIT her forward to ease breathing

Recognizing asthma • *Difficulty breathing often accompanied by coughing* • *Wheezing on* **breathing out** • *Distress and anxiety* • *Fatigue from labored breathing* • *Bluish tinge to face and lips*

1 Ensure the room is well ventilated and smoke-free.

IF *it is a first attack,*
Ⓒ CALL A DOCTOR
IF *the attack is severe or does not respond to medication,*
☎ CALL 911

OR

SIT her on your lap

2 Help your child relax. Sit her down with her arms resting on a table or sit her on your lap. Reassure her since she will be frightened.

IF *your child has special medication, use it early in any attack; see below.*

45

Taking medication

If your child has medication, let him use it. Follow the directions carefully. The attack should ease. If it does not,
☎ CALL 911

Various types of medication are prescribed. Educate your child about his medication so that he knows how to use it when he has an attack.

HELP him to use his inhaler and spacer, if he has one

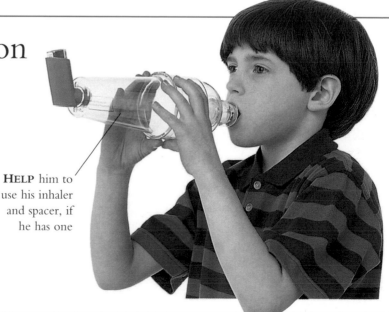

BLEEDING

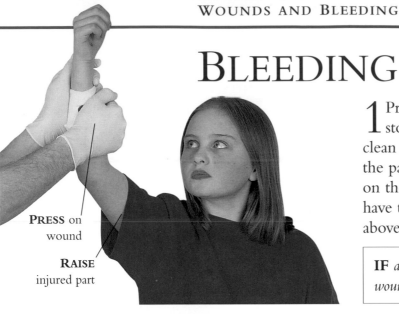

PRESS on
wound

RAISE
injured part

1 Press *firmly* on the wound to
stop the bleeding. Press over a
clean pad or handkerchief or put
the palm of your hand directly
on the wound, using gloves if you
have them. Raise the injured part
above the level of the child's heart.

> **IF** *an object has become stuck in the
> wound, see EMBEDDED OBJECT, p. 48.*

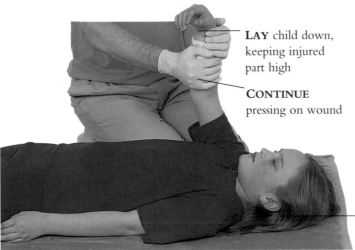

LAY child down,
keeping injured
part high

CONTINUE
pressing on wound

2 Lay your child down, with her
head low (put a thin pad under
her head for comfort), and keep
the injured part raised above the
heart. Keep pressing on the wound
for five minutes.

KEEP her head low – use
a thin pad for comfort

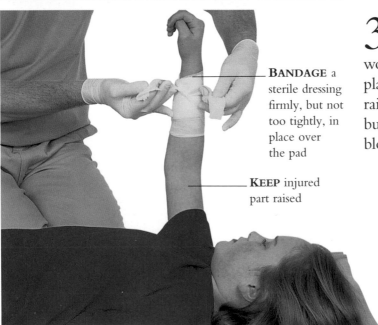

BANDAGE a
sterile dressing
firmly, but not
too tightly, in
place over
the pad

KEEP injured
part raised

3 Cover the wound with a sterile
dressing that is larger than the
wound. Bandage the dressing in
place, still keeping the injured part
raised. The bandage should be firm,
but not so tight as to cut off the
blood supply.

> **IF** *blood comes through the
> bandage, bandage another pad
> firmly on top. If blood continues
> to seep through, remove both
> dressings and apply new ones,
> making sure pressure is applied
> over the wound.*

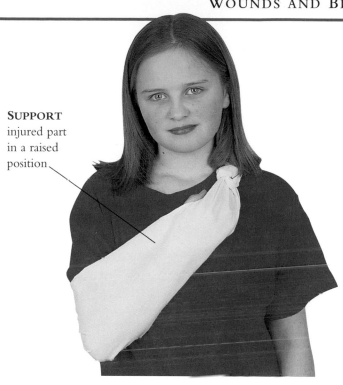

SUPPORT injured part in a raised position

4 When the bleeding is under control, support the injury – for example, with an elevation sling (see p.111).

✚ TAKE YOUR CHILD TO THE HOSPITAL OR ℭ CALL A DOCTOR

> **IF** *the bleeding persists, follow the treatment for* SHOCK, *below.*
> ☎ CALL 911

47

Shock

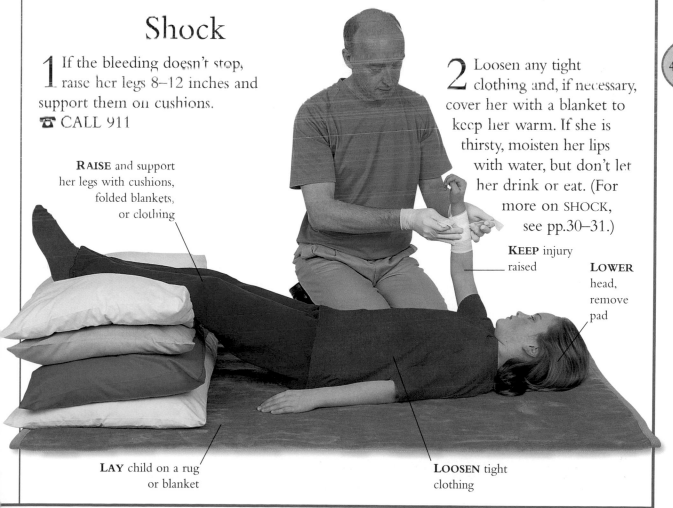

1 If the bleeding doesn't stop, raise her legs 8–12 inches and support them on cushions.
☎ CALL 911

RAISE and support her legs with cushions, folded blankets, or clothing

2 Loosen any tight clothing and, if necessary, cover her with a blanket to keep her warm. If she is thirsty, moisten her lips with water, but don't let her drink or eat. (For more on SHOCK, see pp.30–31.)

KEEP injury raised

LOWER head, remove pad

LAY child on a rug or blanket

LOOSEN tight clothing

EMBEDDED OBJECT

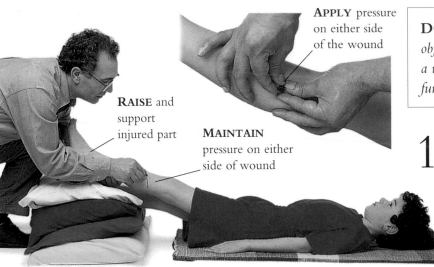

APPLY pressure on either side of the wound

RAISE and support injured part

MAINTAIN pressure on either side of wound

DO NOT *try to remove objects that are embedded in a wound since you may cause further damage and bleeding.*

1 Calm your child and lay her down. Apply pressure on either side of the object and raise the injured part above the level of her heart.

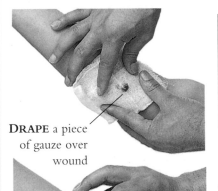

DRAPE a piece of gauze over wound

THIS *advanced technique should be performed by the rescuer only if emergency medical services are unavailable or hours away.*

2 Place a piece of gauze over the wound and object to minimize the risk of infection.

3 Use spare bandage rolls to build up padding to the same height as the embedded object.

PLACE padding around the object

4 Secure the padding by bandaging over it, being careful not to press on the embedded object.
☎ CALL 911

BANDAGE over padding

Bandaging around larger objects

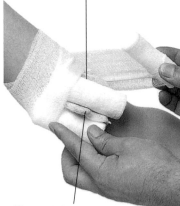

PROTECT object with pads

BANDAGE around object

IF *the object is very big, build padding around it and bandage above and below object.*

48

CUTS AND SCRAPES

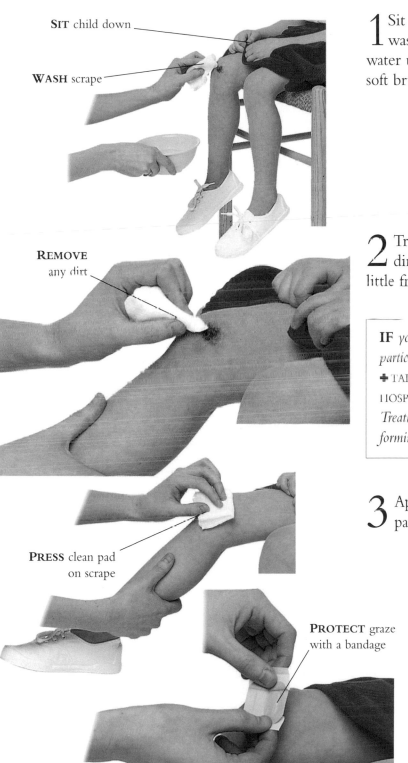

SIT child down

WASH scrape

REMOVE any dirt

PRESS clean pad on scrape

PROTECT graze with a bandage

1 Sit your child down and gently wash the scrape with soap and water using a gauze pad or a very soft brush.

2 Try to remove any particles of dirt or gravel. This may cause a little fresh bleeding.

> **IF** *you cannot remove embedded particles of dirt,*
> ✚ TAKE YOUR CHILD TO THE HOSPITAL
> *Treatment will prevent a tattoo effect forming when the wound heals.*

3 Apply pressure with a clean pad to stop bleeding.

4 Dress the cut or scrape with a bandage that has a pad large enough to cover the wound and the area around it.

> **DO NOT** *cover cuts with cotton, or any fluffy material that may stick to the wound and delay healing.*

49

INFECTED WOUND

Recognizing an infected wound • *Increasing pain and soreness* • *Swelling, redness, and a feeling of heat around the injury* • *Pus within, or oozing from, the wound* • *Swelling and tenderness of glands in the neck, armpit, or groin* • *Faint red trails on the skin leading to these glands.* When infection is advanced • *Feverish signs of sweating, thirst, shivering, and lethargy*

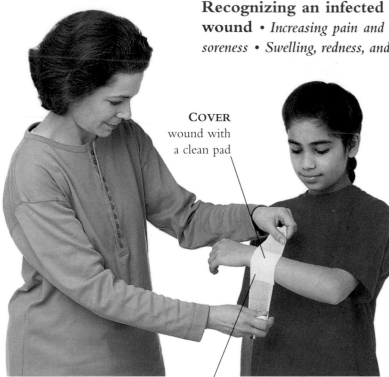

COVER wound with a clean pad

BANDAGE it in place

RAISE and support injury

1 Clean the wound by soaking it in water and washing with soap.

2 Cover the wound with a clean non-fluffy pad or sterile dressing and then bandage it in place.

3 Raise and support the infected wound, for example with an ELEVATION SLING (see p.111).

✆ CALL A DOCTOR OR ✚ TAKE YOUR CHILD TO THE HOSPITAL

TETANUS *is a dangerous infection that is carried in the air or in the soil. Once present in a wound, tetanus germs release toxins (poisons) into the nervous system. It is best prevented through vaccination. Babies receive this as part of their immunization program and a booster is given before starting school.*

50

BLISTERS

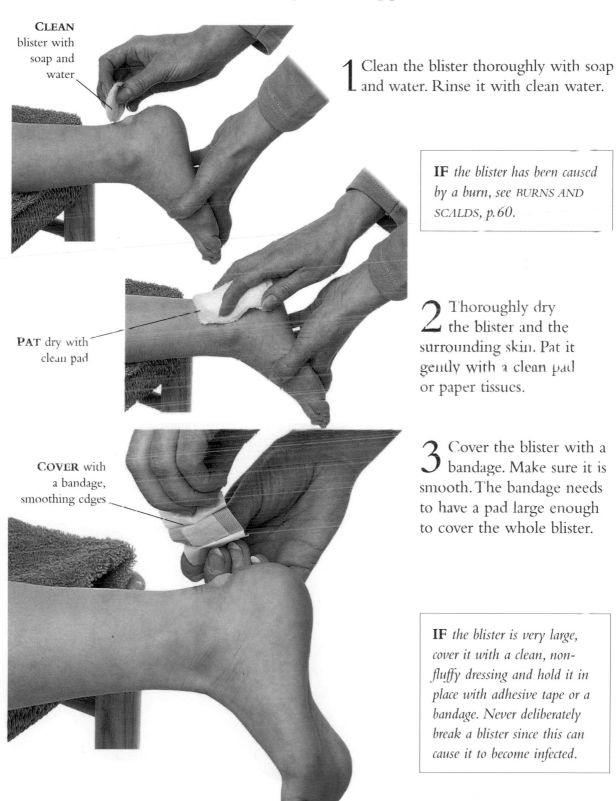

CLEAN blister with soap and water

1 Clean the blister thoroughly with soap and water. Rinse it with clean water.

IF *the blister has been caused by a burn, see* BURNS AND SCALDS, *p.60.*

PAT dry with clean pad

2 Thoroughly dry the blister and the surrounding skin. Pat it gently with a clean pad or paper tissues.

51

COVER with a bandage, smoothing edges

3 Cover the blister with a bandage. Make sure it is smooth. The bandage needs to have a pad large enough to cover the whole blister.

IF *the blister is very large, cover it with a clean, non-fluffy dressing and hold it in place with adhesive tape or a bandage. Never deliberately break a blister since this can cause it to become infected.*

EYE INJURY

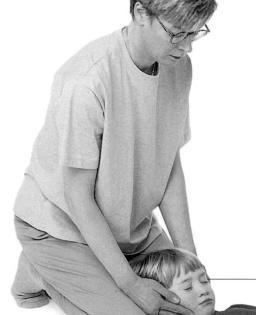

> **FOR** *FOREIGN OBJECT IN THE EYE see p.86.*
> *Do not attempt to remove the object.*
> **FOR** *CHEMICAL BURNS TO THE EYE see p.64.*

1 Lay your child down and cradle his head in your lap to keep it still. Tell him to try not to move his eyes.

TELL him to keep both eyes still

LAY the child down

KEEP his head supported

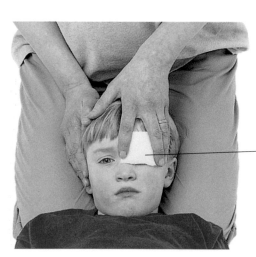

2 Reassure your child and then cover the injured eye to protect it. Hold the dressing gently in place until you get medical help. Do not press on the eye; you may cause further damage.

COVER injured eye with a sterile dressing

> ☎ CALL 911 OR
> ✚ TAKE YOUR CHILD TO THE HOSPITAL
> *Keep him lying on his back.*

52

NOSEBLEED

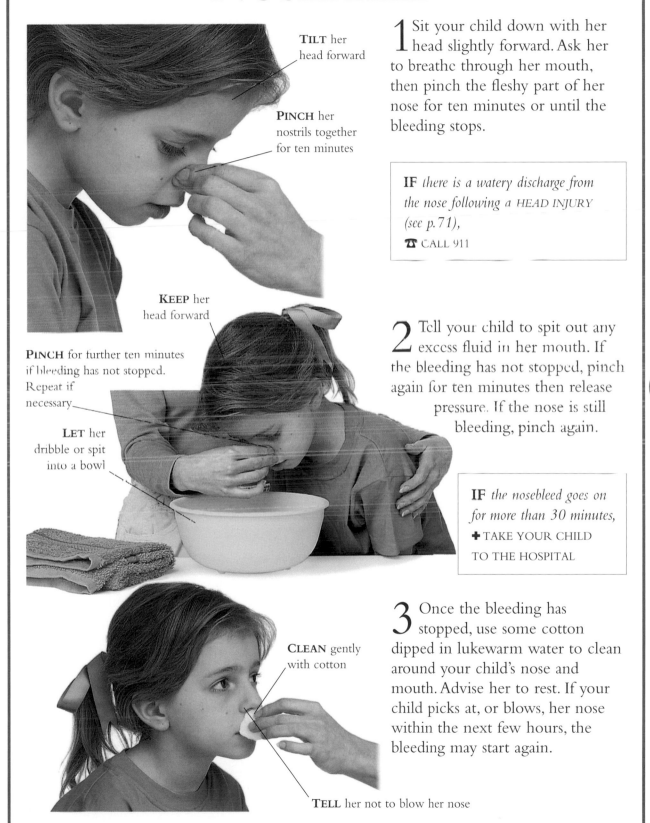

TILT her head forward

PINCH her nostrils together for ten minutes

KEEP her head forward

PINCH for further ten minutes if bleeding has not stopped. Repeat if necessary

LET her dribble or spit into a bowl

CLEAN gently with cotton

TELL her not to blow her nose

1 Sit your child down with her head slightly forward. Ask her to breathe through her mouth, then pinch the fleshy part of her nose for ten minutes or until the bleeding stops.

> **IF** *there is a watery discharge from the nose following a* HEAD INJURY *(see p.71),*
> ☎ CALL 911

2 Tell your child to spit out any excess fluid in her mouth. If the bleeding has not stopped, pinch again for ten minutes then release pressure. If the nose is still bleeding, pinch again.

> **IF** *the nosebleed goes on for more than 30 minutes,*
> ✚ TAKE YOUR CHILD TO THE HOSPITAL

3 Once the bleeding has stopped, use some cotton dipped in lukewarm water to clean around your child's nose and mouth. Advise her to rest. If your child picks at, or blows, her nose within the next few hours, the bleeding may start again.

53

EAR

Bleeding from inside the ear

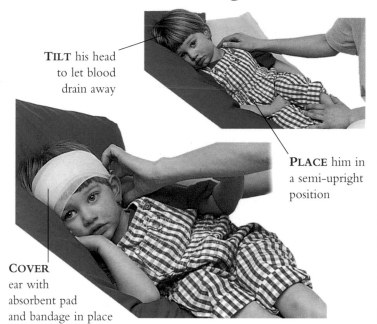

TILT his head to let blood drain away

PLACE him in a semi-upright position

COVER ear with absorbent pad and bandage in place

1 Help your child into a semi-upright position, with his head tilted toward the injured side, to allow blood to drain away.

2 Put an absorbent pad over the ear and bandage it lightly in place. Do not plug the ear.

✆ CALL A DOCTOR

> **IF** *the bleeding follows a head injury (see p.71) and the fluid draining from the ear is thin and watery, keep your child still and try not to move him.*
> ☎ CALL 911

External bleeding

1 Gently pinch the wound with a piece of gauze, pressing for ten minutes.

2 Cover her ear with a sterile dressing and lightly bandage it in place.

✆ CALL A DOCTOR

PRESS on wound over a piece of gauze for ten minutes

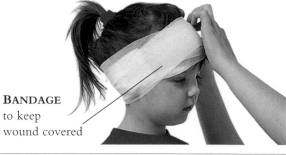

BANDAGE to keep wound covered

> **IF** *the injury is caused by an earring being ripped out or if the ear has been cut, your child may need stitches.*
> ✚ TAKE YOUR CHILD TO THE HOSPITAL

MOUTH INJURY

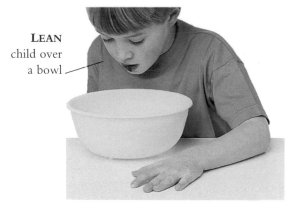

LEAN child over a bowl

DO NOT *wash out his mouth because this may disturb a blood clot.*

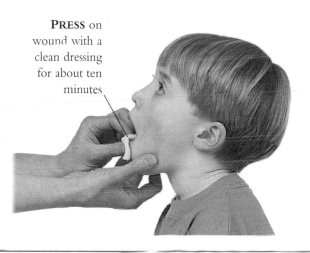

PRESS on wound with a clean dressing for about ten minutes

1 Sit your child down, with his head over a bowl into which he can dribble the blood.

2 Place a dressing over the wound and pinch it between your thumb and forefinger, maintaining the pressure for about ten minutes.

Knocked-out tooth

55

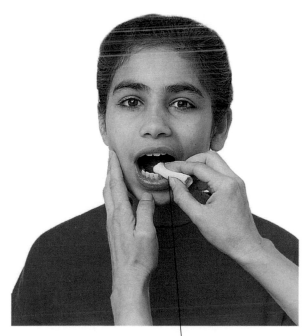

HOLD a dressing over the tooth socket

AN "ADULT" TOOTH *may be reimplanted (put back into place) if it is done soon after the accident. Do not clean the tooth. Put it in milk.*
✚ TAKE YOUR CHILD TO THE DENTIST OR THE HOSPITAL

1 Place a dressing over the tooth socket, making sure that it is higher than the adjacent teeth so that your child can bite on it.

2 Ask your child to sit down with her hand supporting her jaw. Tell her to bite hard on the dressing. A younger child may need you to hold the dressing in place.

BABY TEETH *are not reimplanted, but try to find the tooth to ensure that it has not been inhaled or swallowed. A dentist should check the gum.*

AMPUTATION

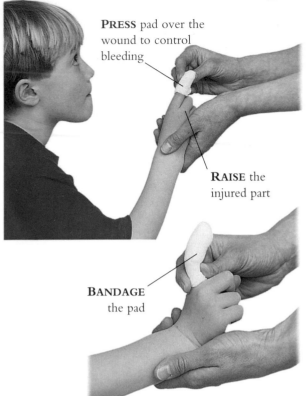

PRESS pad over the wound to control bleeding

RAISE the injured part

BANDAGE the pad

1 Control the blood loss by pressing *firmly* on the injury using a sterile dressing or clean pad. Raise the injured part above the level of your child's heart.

> **DO NOT** *use a tourniquet.*

2 Bandage or tape the dressing firmly in place. You can cover a finger with a gauze finger bandage.

☎ CALL 911
Tell the dispatcher it is an amputation.

> **YOU** *may need to treat your child for* SHOCK, *see p.30, and* BLEEDING, *p.46.*

Care of the amputated part

IT *is often possible to reattach an amputated part using microsurgery. The sooner both the child and the severed part reach the hospital, the better.* **NEVER** *wash the severed part or allow it to come into direct contact with the ice.* **DO NOT** *apply cotton to any raw surface.*

1 Wrap the severed part in plastic wrap or a plastic bag.

2 Wrap the bag in a soft fabric, such as a cotton handkerchief or gauze.

3 Put a plastic bag filled with ice cubes around the fabric. This helps preserve the severed part.

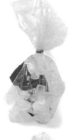

4 Put the whole package in another bag or container. Mark with the time of injury and the child's name. Give it to the ambulance personnel.

INTERNAL BLEEDING

Suspect this when signs of SHOCK (see p.30) develop without obvious blood loss.

Recognizing internal bleeding • *Pale, cold, and sweaty skin tinged with gray* • *A rapid pulse becoming weaker* • *Shallow, fast breathing* • *Restlessness, yawning, and sighing* • *Thirst* • *Possible loss of consciousness.*

After violent injury, there may be: • *"Pattern bruising" at the site of injury with marks from* *clothes or crushing objects* • *Pain* • *Bleeding from orifices — note what it looks like and try to take a sample to the hospital.*

> **IF** *your child loses consciousness, assess her condition (see UNCONSCIOUS BABY, p.16; UNCONSCIOUS CHILD, p.22). Be prepared to resuscitate. If breathing, place her in the RECOVERY POSITION.*

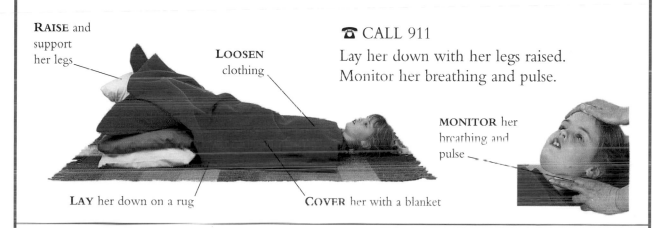

RAISE and support her legs

LOOSEN clothing

LAY her down on a rug

COVER her with a blanket

☎ CALL 911

Lay her down with her legs raised. Monitor her breathing and pulse.

MONITOR her breathing and pulse

57

CRUSH INJURY

☎ CALL 911

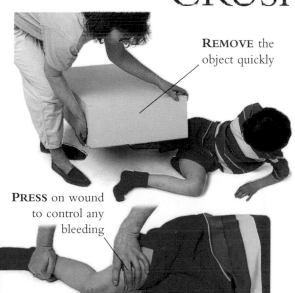

REMOVE the object quickly

PRESS on wound to control any bleeding

> **IF** *the child has been crushed for more than 15 minutes, do not remove the object since this increases the risk of shock and further internal injury. Reassure him.*

1 If the accident has just happened, remove the heavy object immediately.

2 Control any bleeding by pressing firmly on the wound, with your hand or a clean pad.

> **IF** *you suspect broken bones or a head or neck injury, support the injury with padding, but do not move the child until help arrives. Watch for signs of SHOCK (see above and p.30).*

CHEST WOUND

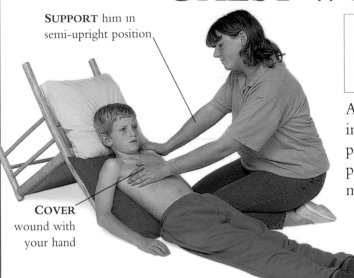

SUPPORT him in semi-upright position

COVER wound with your hand

THIS advanced technique should be performed by the rescuer only if emergency medical services are unavailable or hours away.

A chest wound may cause severe internal damage. The lungs are particularly vulnerable, and breathing problems, shock, and collapsed lungs may follow an injury.

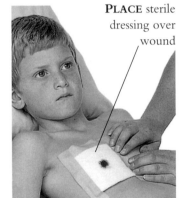

PLACE sterile dressing over wound

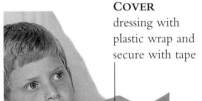

COVER dressing with plastic wrap and secure with tape

☎ CALL 911

1 Cover the wound with the palm of your hand and support your child in a semiupright position.

2 With your child supported, cover the wound with a sterile dressing and tape it in place.

3 Create a seal over the wound with plastic wrap, secured in place with adhesive tape. Leave one corner untaped to permit exhaled air to escape.

4 Incline your child toward his injured side, supported on cushions.

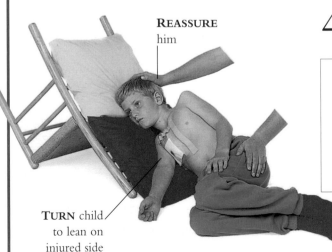

REASSURE him

TURN child to lean on injured side

IF your child loses consciousness, assess his condition (see UNCONSCIOUS BABY, p.16; UNCONSCIOUS CHILD, p.22). Be prepared to resuscitate. If breathing, place him in the RECOVERY POSITION lying on his injured side. Check for signs of SHOCK (see p.30).

58

ABDOMINAL WOUND

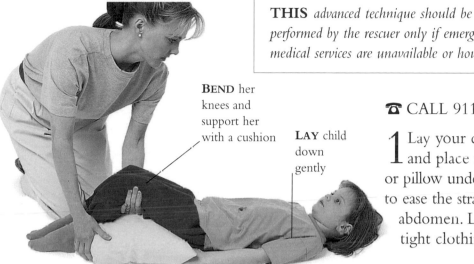

THIS *advanced technique should be performed by the rescuer only if emergency medical services are unavailable or hours away.*

BEND her knees and support her with a cushion

LAY child down gently

☎ CALL 911

1 Lay your child down and place a cushion or pillow under her knees to ease the strain on her abdomen. Loosen any tight clothing.

COVER wound with dressing

2 Reassure your child while you place a large sterile dressing over the wound. Apply pressure over the wound if your child is about to cough or vomit.

IF *part of the intestine is showing, cover it with a polyethylene bag or plastic wrap before dressing the wound.*

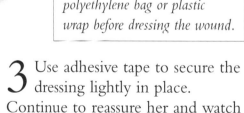

TAPE dressing in place

3 Use adhesive tape to secure the dressing lightly in place. Continue to reassure her and watch for any change in her condition; look particularly for signs of SHOCK (p.30).

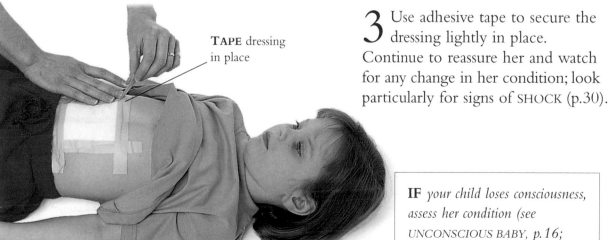

IF *your child loses consciousness, assess her condition (see* UNCONSCIOUS BABY, *p.16;* UNCONSCIOUS CHILD, *p.22). Be prepared to resuscitate.*

BURNS AND SCALDS

For information on dealing with fires, see
ACTION IN AN EMERGENCY p.11.

DO NOT *remove any clothing or material that may be sticking to the burned area because this may cause further damage to the skin.*

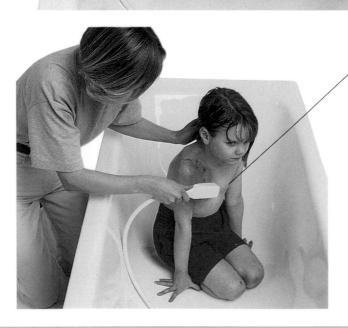

COOL burn with cold water for at least ten minutes

✚ TAKE YOUR CHILD
TO THE HOSPITAL
OR
☎ CALL 911

1 To stop the burning process and relieve pain, cool the burn with cold water for at least ten minutes.

IF *no cold water is available, use another cool liquid, such as milk.*

DO NOT *immerse young children in cold water because this can cause hypothermia.*

REMOVE cooled clothing and cool injury again

2 Once cooled, remove clothing from the burned area and, if the pain persists, cool again. Cut around any material that is sticking to the skin. Remove all restrictive clothing from the area of a burn before any swelling occurs.

DO NOT *touch the burn or burst any blisters.*

60

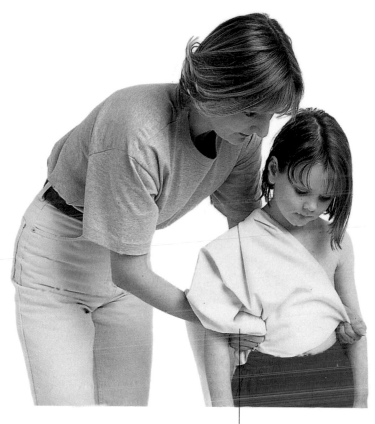

3 Cover the burn with clean, nonfluffy material to protect it from infection. You can use a clean sheet or pillowcase. The dressing does not need to be secured. Do not apply lotions, fat, or ointment. Ensure that your child remains warm to prevent the onset of hypothermia.

DO NOT *give her anything to eat or drink and watch for signs of* SHOCK *(see p. 30).*

IF *she loses consciousness, assess her condition (see* UNCONSCIOUS BABY, *p. 16;* UNCONSCIOUS CHILD, *p. 22). Be prepared to resuscitate. If breathing, place her in the* RECOVERY POSITION *(p. 24).*

COVER burn loosely with clean, nonfluffy material

Alternative dressings

To dress a burned hand or foot you can use a plastic bag, which will protect the burn from infection. Secure the bag with a bandage or tape around the bag, not the skin.

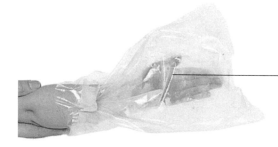

PROTECT with clean plastic bag

Burns to the mouth and throat

Burns in this area are very serious since they cause swelling and inflammation of the air passages, giving a serious risk of suffocation. Act quickly. If necessary, loosen clothing from around his neck.

☎ CALL 911

IF *your child develops breathing difficulties, assess his condition (see* UNCONSCIOUS BABY, *p. 16;* UNCONSCIOUS CHILD, *p. 22). Be prepared to resuscitate.*

61

ELECTRICAL BURN

An electric shock from a low-voltage source can result in burns. These may occur at both the point of entry and the point of exit of an electrical current. See ELECTRICAL INJURY (p.12), SHOCK (p.30).

> **DO NOT** *touch your child directly until you are sure the electrical current is switched off.*

> **IF** *your child loses consciousness, assess her condition (see UNCONSCIOUS BABY, p.16; UNCONSCIOUS CHILD, p.22). Be prepared to resuscitate. If breathing, place her in the RECOVERY POSITION (see p.24).*

COOL burns with cold water for at least ten minutes

1 Hold the injured area under cold, running water for at least ten minutes to cool the burn.

2 Protect the burn by covering it with clean, smooth material or with a plastic bag, held or taped in place.

+ TAKE YOUR CHILD TO THE HOSPITAL

COVER with a clean plastic bag

62

CHEMICAL BURN TO SKIN

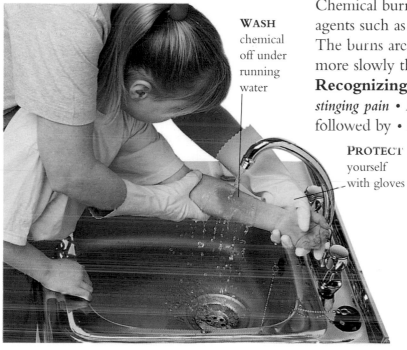

WASH chemical off under running water

PROTECT yourself with gloves

Chemical burns can be caused by household agents such as oven cleaner or paint stripper. The burns are serious but signs develop more slowly than for thermal burns.
Recognizing chemical burns • *Fierce, stinging pain* • *Redness or skin discoloration,* followed by • *Blistering and peeling*

1 Wash away all traces of the chemical by holding the affected area under plenty of cool running water.

> **NOTE** *the name of the substance that caused the burn. Wear protective rubber gloves, and beware of fumes. See* SMOKE INHALATION, *p. 43, and* SWALLOWED CHEMICALS, *p. 65.*

63

Removing clothes

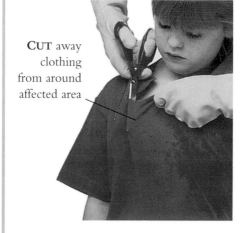

CUT away clothing from around affected area

Cut off clothing from the affected area, unless you can slip it off without touching other parts of the body. Avoid cutting through the affected area – cut around it instead.

COVER burn loosely with clean, smooth material

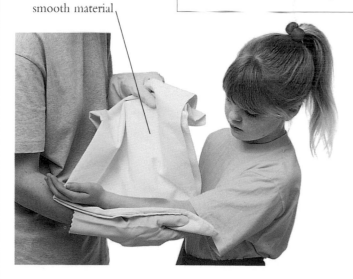

2 Loosely cover the burn with clean, smooth material to avoid constriction when the wound swells. You can wet the material to cool the burn.

✚ TAKE YOUR CHILD TO THE HOSPITAL OR
☎ CALL 911

CHEMICAL BURN TO EYE

Splashes of chemicals in the eye can cause scarring or can even cause blindness.

Recognizing chemical burns to the eye • *Fierce pain in the eye* • *Difficulty opening the eye* • *Redness and swelling in and around the eye* • *Very watery eye*

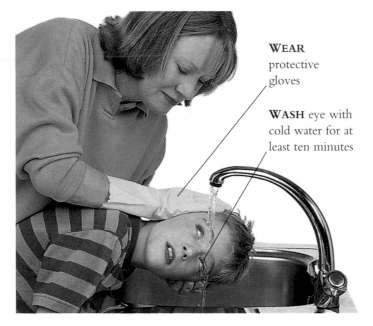

WEAR protective gloves

WASH eye with cold water for at least ten minutes

DO NOT *let your child touch his eye.*

THE EYE *will be shut in spasm and pain, so gently pull the eyelids open.*

1 Hold your child's head over a sink or basin, with the "good" eye uppermost. Gently run cold water over the contaminated eye for at least ten minutes. Wear protective gloves. Make sure that both sides of the eyelid are thoroughly washed and that the water drains away from his face.

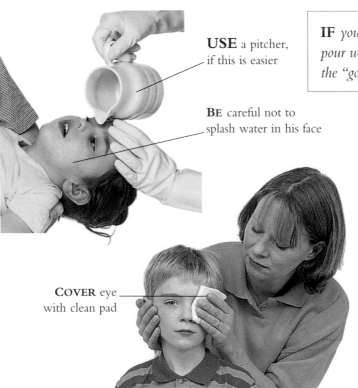

USE a pitcher, if this is easier

BE careful not to splash water in his face

IF *you find it easier, you can use a pitcher to pour water over the affected eye. Avoid splashing the "good" eye with contaminated water.*

---

2 When the injured eye is thoroughly washed, cover it with a protective device like the top of a paper cup. Do not press on the eye.

✚ TAKE YOUR CHILD TO THE HOSPITAL
OR
☎ CALL 911

COVER eye with clean pad

SWALLOWED CHEMICALS

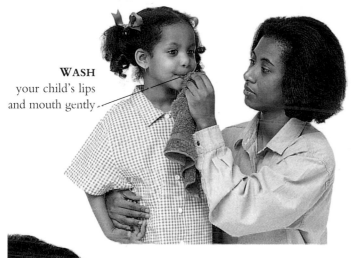

WASH your child's lips and mouth gently

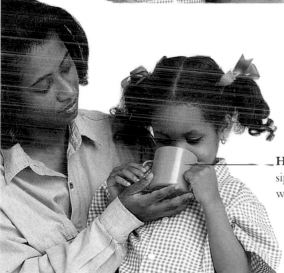

IF *you think your child has swallowed anything poisonous,* ☠ CALL YOUR LOCAL POISON CONTROL CENTER OR 1-800-268-9017

1 Wipe away any residual chemical around the mouth and face.

2 Her lips may be burned or discolored. Give her frequent sips of cold water or milk, but only if told to do so by the doctor or the poison control center.

HELP her take sips of cold water or milk

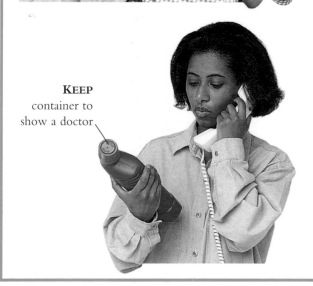

DO NOT *try to make your child vomit since this can cause further harm.*

3 Find out what chemical your child swallowed and telephone a doctor or the poison control center with the information. This will help determine the correct medical treatment.

KEEP container to show a doctor

IF *your child loses consciousness, assess her condition (see UNCONSCIOUS BABY, p. 16; UNCONSCIOUS CHILD, p. 22). Be prepared to resuscitate. If breathing, place her in the RECOVERY POSITION (p. 24).*

65

DRUG POISONING

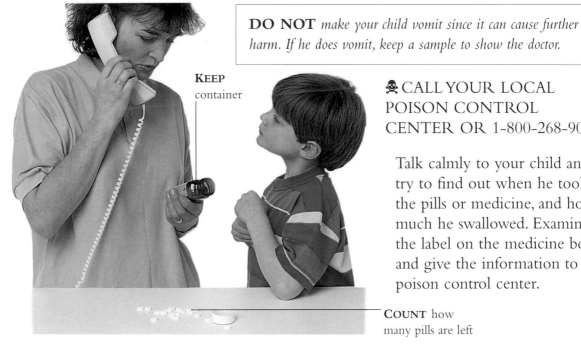

DO NOT *make your child vomit since it can cause further harm. If he does vomit, keep a sample to show the doctor.*

KEEP container

☠ CALL YOUR LOCAL POISON CONTROL CENTER OR 1-800-268-9017

Talk calmly to your child and try to find out when he took the pills or medicine, and how much he swallowed. Examine the label on the medicine bottle and give the information to the poison control center.

COUNT how many pills are left

If the child is unconscious

☎ CALL 911

CLEAR his mouth, if necessary

1 Open his mouth. Pick out any drugs that you can see.

TRY *to find out what drugs he has taken and how much he has swallowed.*

OPEN airway

CHECK for breathing

2 Open his airway. Check his breathing (see UNCONSCIOUS BABY, p.16; UNCONSCIOUS CHILD, p.22). Be prepared to resuscitate. If he is breathing, place him in the RECOVERY POSITION (p.24). Stay with him until help arrives.

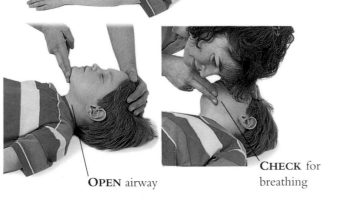

PLACE him in recovery position if breathing

66

ALCOHOL POISONING

> **EVEN** *a small amount of alcohol may harm a young child.*

QUESTION her calmly

LOOK for symptoms of alcohol poisoning

EXAMINE bottle to see how much she has drunk

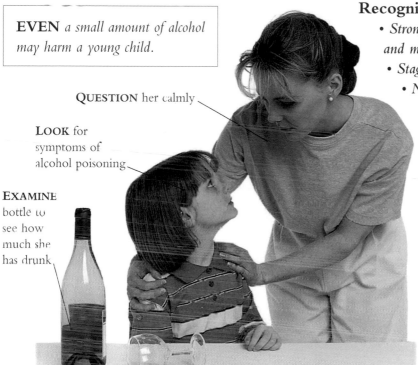

Recognizing alcohol poisoning
- Strong smell of alcohol • Flushed and moist face • Slurred speech
- • Staggering • Deep noisy breathing
- • Nausea • Bounding pulse

☎ CALL A DOCTOR

Allow your child to rest where you can watch over her. Place a bowl nearby in case she vomits. If she falls asleep, check her to make sure she can be easily roused. If she is very drowsy, or seems unconscious, see below.

67

If the child is unconscious

☎ CALL 911

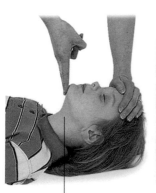

OPEN airway

CHECK for breathing

> **KEEP** *your child warm. Alcohol dilates the blood vessels, which can cause hypothermia.*

Open her airway. Check her breathing (see UNCONSCIOUS BABY, p.16; UNCONSCIOUS CHILD, p.22). Be prepared to resuscitate. If she is breathing, place her in the RECOVERY POSITION (p.24). Stay with her until help arrives.

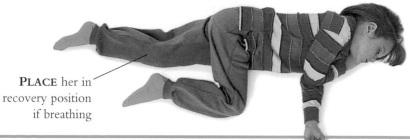

PLACE her in recovery position if breathing

PLANT POISONING

> **DO NOT** *make your child vomit. This can cause further harm. If he does vomit, show a sample to the doctor.*

1 Try to find out what your child has eaten and keep a sample to show the doctor.
☠ CALL YOUR LOCAL POISON CONTROL CENTER OR 1-800-268-9017

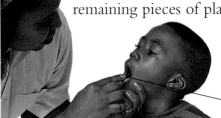

2 Look inside your child's mouth Using your fingers, pick out any remaining pieces of plant or berries.

KEEP piece of plant or any berries to show doctor

REMOVE any residue

If the child is unconscious

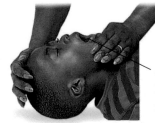

1 Open his mouth. Pick out any pieces of plant that you can see.
☎ CALL 911

CLEAR his mouth if necessary

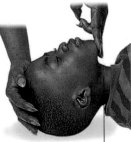

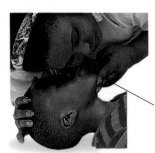

2 Open his airway. Check his breathing (see UNCONSCIOUS BABY, p.16; UNCONSCIOUS CHILD, p.22). Be prepared to resuscitate.

CHECK for breathing

OPEN airway

> **IF** *he is breathing, place him in the RECOVERY POSITION (see p.24). Stay with him until the ambulance arrives.*

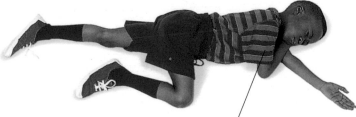

PLACE him in recovery position if breathing

SCALP AND FOREHEAD WOUND

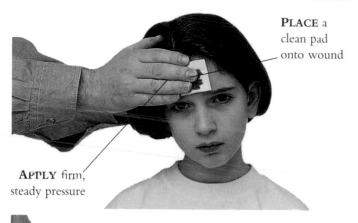

PLACE a clean pad onto wound

APPLY firm, steady pressure

1 Cover the injury with a clean pad or sterile dressing that is larger than the wound. Press firmly on the pad and the wound to control the bleeding. Place another pad on top, if necessary, and keep pressing on the wound. If blood continues to seep through, remove both pads and apply new ones.

BANDAGE pad in place

SECURE bandage firmly but not too tightly

2 Bandage the dressing firmly in place. If the bleeding continues, apply pressure again with your hand.

> **IF** *the wound has been caused by a blow to the head,*
> ☏ CALL A DOCTOR
> *(see also CONCUSSION p.70; SKULL FRACTURE p.71).*

69

3 Help your child to lie down with her head and shoulders slightly raised. Watch for any changes.

☎ CALL 911 OR
✚ TAKE HER TO THE HOSPITAL

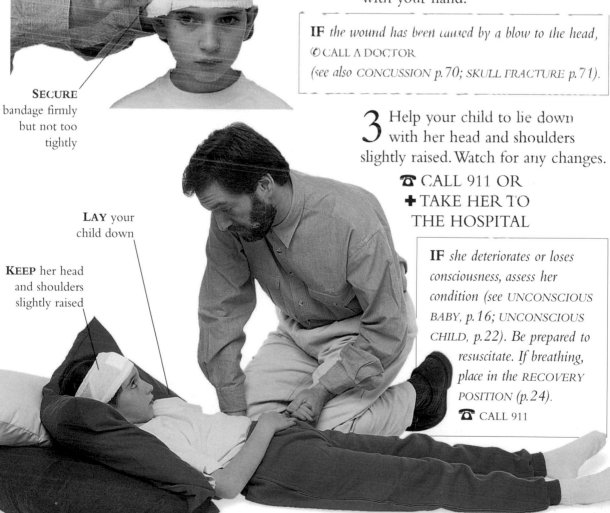

LAY your child down

KEEP her head and shoulders slightly raised

> **IF** *she deteriorates or loses consciousness, assess her condition (see UNCONSCIOUS BABY, p.16; UNCONSCIOUS CHILD, p.22). Be prepared to resuscitate. If breathing, place in the RECOVERY POSITION (p.24).*
> ☎ CALL 911

CONCUSSION

The brain may be "shaken" by a blow causing concussion. The period of unconsciousness is brief and followed by complete recovery. You should be able to distinguish between a bump on the head with no concussion, a brief period of unconsciousness (less than 20 seconds), and an extended period of unconsciousness.

Recognizing concussion • *Brief loss of consciousness, dizziness or nausea on recovery*
• *Loss of memory of immediately preceding events*
• *A mild headache*

Conscious child

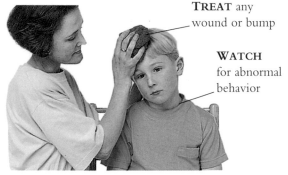

TREAT any wound or bump

WATCH for abnormal behavior

If your child has bumped his head, sit him down and treat any minor bruise or wound with a cold compress.

> **WATCH** *for signs of abnormal behavior. If he does not recover fully within a few minutes,*
> ℂ CALL A DOCTOR

Child who regains consciousness quickly

1 If your child has been "knocked out," even briefly,
ℂ CALL A DOCTOR

2 Make her rest and watch her closely. If she does not recover completely within 30 minutes,
☎ CALL 911

WATCH child carefully for abnormal behavior

MAKE sure she rests

Unconscious child

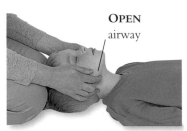

OPEN airway

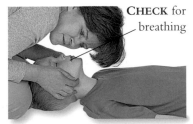

CHECK for breathing

> **IF** *you are alone and you need to leave your child to call an ambulance, and if your child remains unconscious, place him in the RECOVERY POSITION (see p.24) before you leave.*

☎ CALL 911

Open your child's airway using the jaw thrust technique (see p.74). Check his breathing (see UNCONSCIOUS BABY, p.16; UNCONSCIOUS CHILD, p.22). Be prepared to resuscitate. If he is breathing, continue to support his head and keep his neck still until help arrives.

SKULL FRACTURE

Fractures of the skull are potentially very serious injuries and require urgent medical attention to minimize the risk of damage to the brain and the possibility of infection.

Recognizing a skull fracture • *Wound or bruise on the head* • *Soft area on the scalp* • *Impaired consciousness* • *Deterioration in level of response* • *Clear fluid from the nose or ear*

• *Blood showing in the white of the eye*
• *Distortion of the head or face*

☎ CALL 911

> **IF** *you suspect BACK or NECK INJURIES, see pp. 73–74.*

Unconscious child

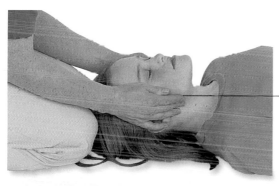

LIFT your child's jaw up with your fingertips

1 Open your child's airway using the jaw thrust technique (see p.74).

> **IF** *you are alone and you need to leave your child to call an ambulance, and if your child remains unconscious, place her in the RECOVERY POSITION (see p.24) before you leave.*

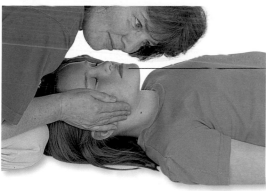

CHECK for breathing

2 Check her breathing (see UNCONSCIOUS BABY, p.16; UNCONSCIOUS CHILD, p.22). Be prepared to resuscitate. If your child is breathing, continue to support her head and keep her neck still until help arrives.

71

Delayed reaction

There may be a serious reaction to a head injury hours later. Brain edema (swelling) is a condition caused by blood accumulating within the skull and putting pressure on the brain.

Recognizing brain edema (swelling)
• *Disorientation and confusion* • *Severe headache*

• *Impaired consciousness* • *Noisy breathing, becoming slow* • *Slow but strong pulse* • *Unequal pupils* • *Weakness or paralysis* • *Raised temperature*

Be prepared to resuscitate (see UNCONSCIOUS BABY, p.16; UNCONSCIOUS CHILD, p.22).

☎ CALL 911

BROKEN NOSE/CHEEKBONE

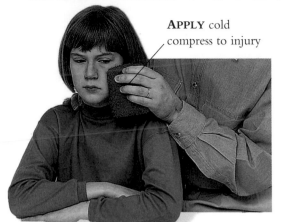

APPLY cold compress to injury

1 Sit your child down and apply a cold compress to the injured part. This helps to reduce the swelling. Hold the compress in place for about 30 minutes.

2 If your child's nose is bleeding heavily, ask her to sit with her head over a bowl and to pinch her nostrils together.

PINCH nostrils together to stop bleeding

SIT your child well forward over bowl

IF *pinching her nose hurts too much, simply ask her to sit forward and give her a soft pad or towel to soak up the blood.*
✚ TAKE YOUR CHILD TO THE HOSPITAL OR
☎ CALL 911

BROKEN JAW

Recognizing a broken jaw
• *Tender, swollen, bruised jaw* • *Teeth may be out of line*

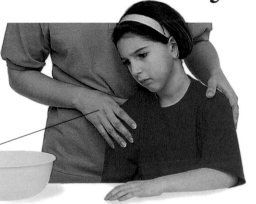

HELP her lean forward

1 Sit her down with her head well forward. Tell her not to swallow, but to let any blood or saliva drain away.

IF *she loses consciousness, assess her condition (see UNCONSCIOUS BABY, p.16; UNCONSCIOUS CHILD, p.22). Be prepared to resuscitate. If breathing, place her in the RECOVERY POSITION.*
☎ CALL 911

HOLD pad against jaw and support jaw with your hand

2 Hold a soft pad firmly under her jaw. Do not bandage it in place in case she vomits. Support the jaw on the way to the hospital.

✚ TAKE YOUR CHILD
TO THE HOSPITAL OR
☎ CALL 911

BACK AND NECK INJURIES
The conscious child

☎ CALL 911

LEAVE a slight gap so that your child can hear you

HOLD his head in your hands

> **DO NOT** *move the injured child unless his life is in danger. If you do have to move him, try to do so in "one piece," taking care not to twist or bend the neck or spine.*

1 Reassure your child and tell him not to move. Steady and support his head and neck in the position in which you found him, by placing your hands over his ears. Be careful not to pull on his neck.

MAINTAIN support of his head

2 Keep his head supported in the position you found him until help arrives. Ask someone to put rolled blankets or towels around his neck and shoulders for extra support.

PLACE rolled blankets around his head and shoulders

CONTINUE to support his head

3 Get your helper to arrange rolled towels or blankets along either side of the child's body while you continue to keep his head and neck steady.

PLACE folded blankets or towels either side of his body

73

BACK AND NECK INJURIES
The unconscious child

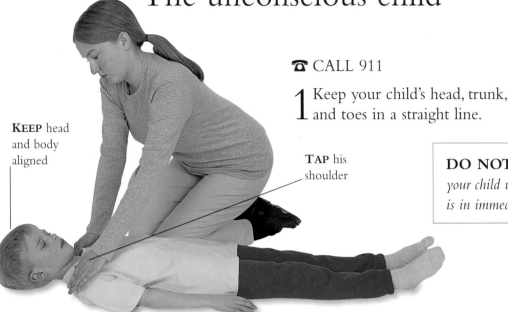

KEEP head and body aligned

TAP his shoulder

☎ CALL 911

1 Keep your child's head, trunk, and toes in a straight line.

> **DO NOT MOVE**
> *your child unless his life is in immediate danger.*

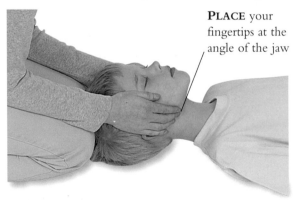

PLACE your fingertips at the angle of the jaw

2 Use the jaw thrust method to open your child's airway. Kneel behind his head and place your hands on both sides of his face, with your fingertips at the angles of his jaw. Gently lift his jaw to open the airway, taking care not to tilt his head back.

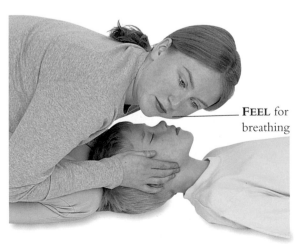

FEEL for breathing

3 Check his breathing (see UNCONSCIOUS BABY, p.16; UNCONSCIOUS CHILD, p.22). Be prepared to resuscitate. If your child is breathing, continue to support his head until help arrives. If you cannot maintain an open airway, place him in the RECOVERY POSITION (see opposite).

> **IF** *you are alone and need to leave your child to call an ambulance, and if your child remains unconscious, place him in the RECOVERY POSITION (see p.24) before you leave.*

Recovery position with one helper

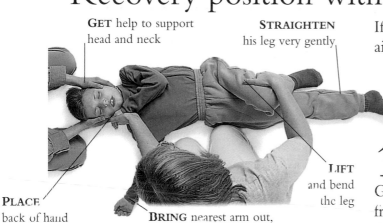

GET help to support head and neck

STRAIGHTEN his leg very gently

LIFT and bend the leg

PLACE back of hand against his cheek

BRING nearest arm out, elbow bent, palm uppermost

If you cannot maintain an open airway, for example if your child vomits, place him in the recovery position. See p.24 if you have no helper.

1 Ask the helper to support your child's head with her hands. Grasp the thigh of the leg farthest from you. Gently lift and bend the leg. Draw the arm farthest from you across the child's chest.

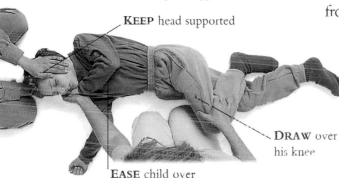

KEEP head supported

DRAW over his knee

EASE child over

2 Draw over his knee and ease him around gently. Keep his head and trunk aligned at all times.

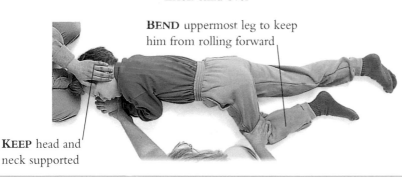

BEND uppermost leg to keep him from rolling forward

KEEP head and neck supported

3 With your child turned onto his side, maintain an open airway and support him in this position until help arrives. Monitor his breathing and pulse. Be prepared to resuscitate (see UNCONSCIOUS BABY, p.16; UNCONSCIOUS CHILD, p.22).

75

Log-roll technique

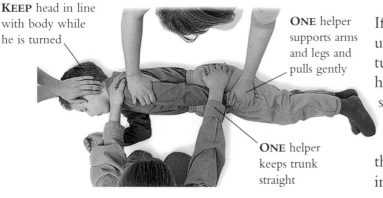

KEEP head in line with body while he is turned

ONE helper supports arms and legs and pulls gently

ONE helper keeps trunk straight

If you have two or more helpers, use the "log-roll" technique to turn your child. It is vital to keep his head, trunk, and feet in a straight line. While one adult holds the child's head, two others should gently straighten the limbs and roll the child over in one synchronized movement.

BROKEN LOWER LEG

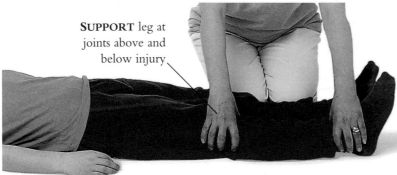

SUPPORT leg at joints above and below injury

1 Lay your child down gently and support his leg at the ankle and knee joints. Ask someone to help you, if possible.

2 Steady the injured leg with padding. Place one rolled-up blanket outside the injured limb and one between the legs. If necessary, cover him with another blanket to keep him warm.

☎ CALL 911

MAKE a J-shaped pad with a rolled blanket and place it around his leg

76

Making binder and cravat bandages

TAKE a triangular bandage

FOLD top point over to touch the base

BINDER BANDAGE

FOLD bandage in half to make a binder bandage

CRAVAT BANDAGE

FOLD bandage in half again to make a cravat bandage

Tying a square knot

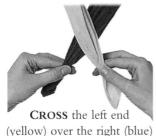

CROSS the left end (yellow) over the right (blue)

TAKE the yellow under and through

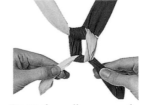

PASS the yellow over the blue and through the gap

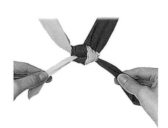

PULL the ends firmly

How to splint an injured leg

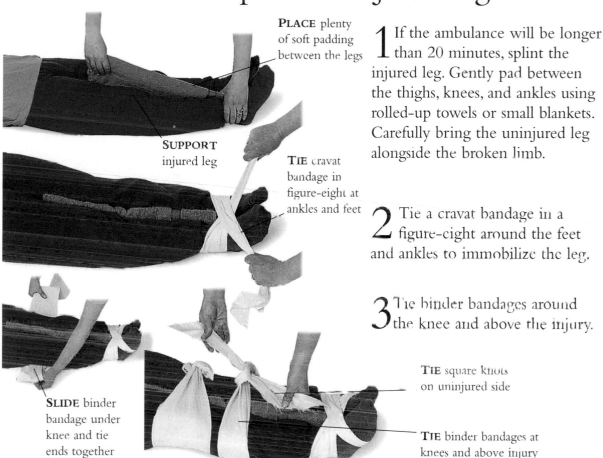

PLACE plenty of soft padding between the legs

SUPPORT injured leg

TIE cravat bandage in figure-eight at ankles and feet

SLIDE binder bandage under knee and tie ends together

TIE square knots on uninjured side

TIE binder bandages at knees and above injury

1 If the ambulance will be longer than 20 minutes, splint the injured leg. Gently pad between the thighs, knees, and ankles using rolled-up towels or small blankets. Carefully bring the uninjured leg alongside the broken limb.

2 Tie a cravat bandage in a figure-eight around the feet and ankles to immobilize the leg.

3 Tie binder bandages around the knee and above the injury.

BROKEN UPPER LEG OR PELVIS

INJURIES *to the pelvis are usually caused by crushing or direct impact. There may be INTERNAL BLEEDING (p.57). SHOCK may develop (p.30).*

☎ CALL 911

Recognizing a broken pelvis
• *Inability to walk or stand*
• *Pain and tenderness in the hip and groin region*
• *Bleeding from the urinary orifice*

Lay your child down gently, keeping her head low. Place padding between her legs. Immobilize the legs with a figure-eight cravat bandage and binder bandages, see above. Placing cushions under the knees may help alleviate pain.

DO NOT *bandage if it causes pain.*

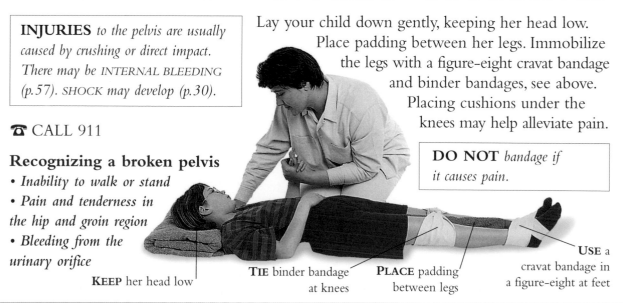

KEEP her head low

TIE binder bandage at knees

PLACE padding between legs

USE a cravat bandage in a figure-eight at feet

77

KNEE INJURY

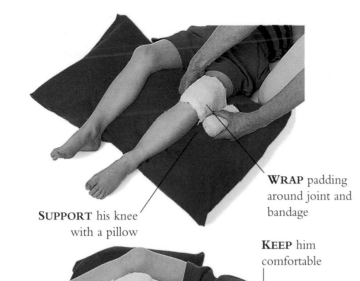

1 Help your child to lie down, then slide a pillow under the injured knee to provide support. Pad around the injured knee with cotton or a soft dressing.

2 Use a roller bandage to keep the padding in place, working from the child's injured side.

WRAP padding around joint and bandage

SUPPORT his knee with a pillow

KEEP him comfortable

> **DO NOT** *attempt to force the knee straight as this may cause further injury.*

> **DO NOT** *allow the child to eat, drink, or walk.*

☎ CALL 911

78

BROKEN FOOT

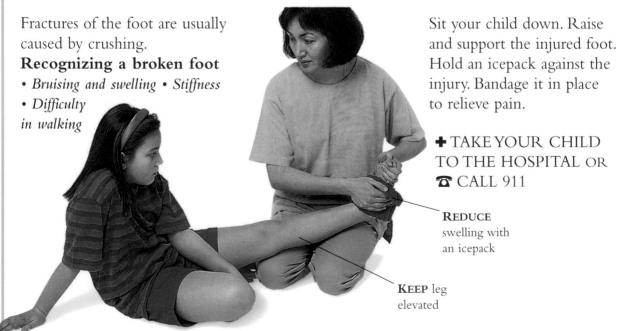

Fractures of the foot are usually caused by crushing.

Recognizing a broken foot
• *Bruising and swelling* • *Stiffness*
• *Difficulty in walking*

Sit your child down. Raise and support the injured foot. Hold an icepack against the injury. Bandage it in place to relieve pain.

✚ TAKE YOUR CHILD TO THE HOSPITAL OR ☎ CALL 911

REDUCE swelling with an icepack

KEEP leg elevated

BROKEN OR SPRAINED ANKLE

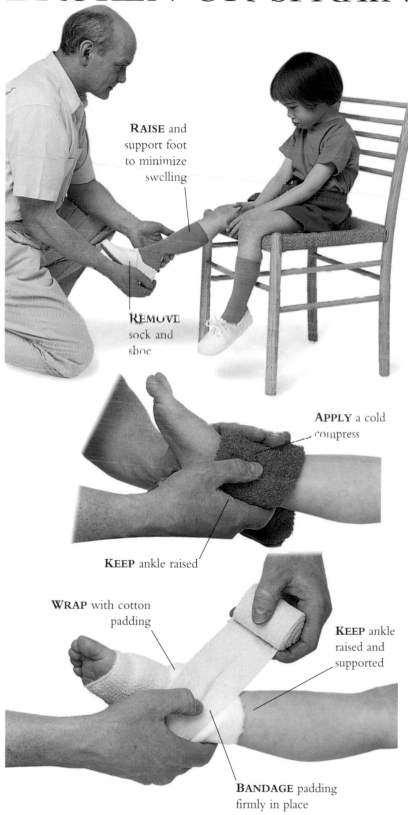

RAISE and support foot to minimize swelling

REMOVE sock and shoe

APPLY a cold compress

KEEP ankle raised

WRAP with cotton padding

KEEP ankle raised and supported

BANDAGE padding firmly in place

Suspect an ankle sprain if your child can't take her full weight on her foot after a fall or twist. Children are more likely to have a fracture than a sprain, since their growing bones are weaker than the ligaments that hold the bones together. (In adults, the ligaments are weaker than the bones.)

1 Sit your child down to rest her foot. Raise her foot and gently remove her sock and shoe before swelling occurs.

2 To minimize swelling, apply a COLD COMPRESS, such as a washcloth wrung out in cold water or an icepack (see p.84).

3 Wrap the ankle with a thick layer of cotton. Bandage cotton firmly in place. Keep the ankle raised.

✆ CALL A DOCTOR OR
☎ CALL 911

IF *you suspect a BROKEN FOOT, see opposite.*
✚ TAKE YOUR CHILD TO THE HOSPITAL

79

BROKEN COLLAR BONE

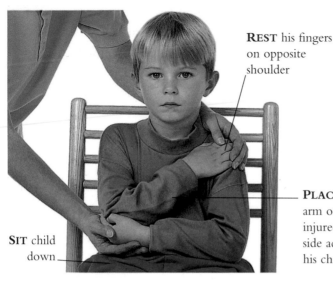

REST his fingers on opposite shoulder

PLACE arm on injured side across his chest

SIT child down

The collar bone may be broken by indirect force, if a child falls onto his outstretched hand, or by a blow to his shoulder.

Recognizing a broken collar bone • *Pain and tenderness increased by movement* • *Head turned and inclined to the injured side*

1 Sit your child down and gently bring the arm on the injured side across his chest. Ask him to support his elbow in his hand.

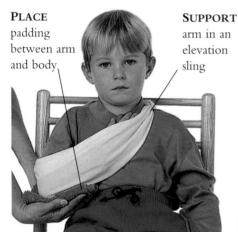

PLACE padding between arm and body

SUPPORT arm in an elevation sling

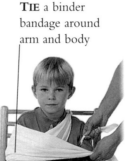

TIE a binder bandage around arm and body

2 Place your child's arm in an ELEVATION SLING for support (see p.111). Use a SQUARE KNOT (see p.76).

3 Secure the arm with a BINDER BANDAGE tied loosely around the body (see p.76 and below).

✚ TAKE YOUR CHILD TO THE HOSPITAL

Tying a binder bandage around a sling

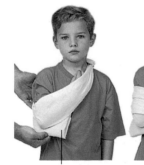

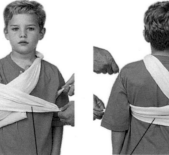

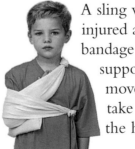

A sling will support an injured arm, but a binder bandage provides extra support and prevents movement when you take your child to the hospital.

SLIDE padding between arm and body

PLACE a binder bandage loosely around body and arm

SECURE with a square knot tied on uninjured side

80

BROKEN RIBS

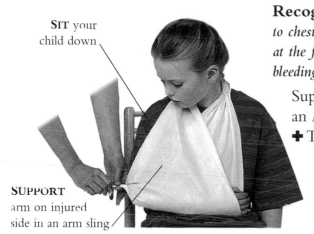

SIT your child down

SUPPORT arm on injured side in an arm sling

Recognizing broken ribs • *Child has had a blow to chest, a heavy fall, or has been crushed* • *Sharp pain at the fracture site* • *Pain on breathing* • *Signs of internal bleeding* • *Open wound over the fracture site*

Support the arm on the injured side in an ARM SLING (see p.110).

✚ TAKE YOUR CHILD TO THE HOSPITAL

> **IF** *the child has a* CHEST WOUND *(see p.58) or* INTERNAL BLEEDING *(see p.57),*
> ☎ CALL 911

Open or multiple rib fractures

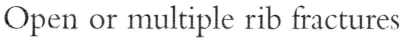

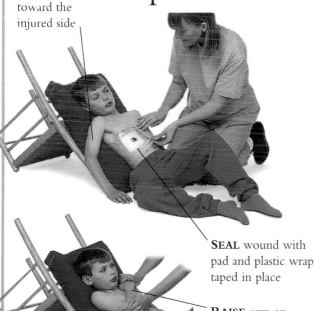

LEAN child toward the injured side

SEAL wound with pad and plastic wrap taped in place

RAISE arm on injured side across his chest

PUT arm on injured side in elevation sling

☎ CALL 911

Treat any open wound and support the chest wall to safeguard breathing (see also CHEST WOUND, p.58).

1 Help the child into a semiupright position supported by pillows. Incline his body toward the injured side. Cover any wounds to the chest wall using a sterile pad. Then seal with plastic wrap. Secure pad on three sides with tape.

2 Place the arm on the injured side across your child's chest.

3 Support the raised arm in an ELEVATION SLING (see p.111). Keep him as comfortable as possible while you wait for the ambulance.

> **IF** *your child loses consciousness or develops breathing difficulties, assess his condition (see* UNCONSCIOUS BABY, *p.16;* UNCONSCIOUS CHILD, *p.22). Be prepared to resuscitate.*

81

BROKEN ARM

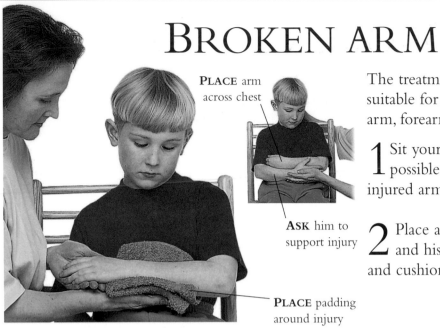

PLACE arm across chest

ASK him to support injury

PLACE padding around injury

SUPPORT arm in a sling

TIE a binder bandage around arm and chest

The treatment described below is suitable for injuries to the upper arm, forearm, and wrist.

1 Sit your child down and if possible get him to support his injured arm in his hand.

2 Place a pad between his arm and his chest to immobilize and cushion the injured limb.

3 Put the injured limb in an ARM SLING (see p.110), secured with a SQUARE KNOT (see p.76).

4 For additional support, place a BINDER BANDAGE over the sling and around your child's arm and chest (see p.76 and 80).

✚ TAKE YOUR CHILD TO THE HOSPITAL

82

BROKEN ELBOW

Elbow injuries need special care and early treatment in the hospital.

Recognizing a broken elbow • *Pain increased by attempted movement* • *Stiffness* • *Swelling or bruising*

> **DO NOT** *attempt to straighten or bend the elbow.*

☎ CALL 911

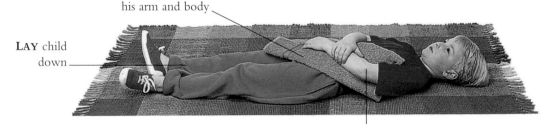

PUT soft padding between his arm and body

LAY child down

PLACE injured arm across his body

BROKEN HAND

WRAP hand in
soft padding

1 Wrap the injured hand in a bulky dressing. Raise your child's hand, supporting it to minimize swelling.

IF *there is a wound, control the bleeding by raising the hand and applying gentle pressure over a clean dressing.*

COVER any wound with a dressing

APPLY pressure to control bleeding

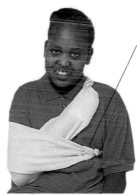

2 Place your child's arm in an ELEVATION SLING (see p.111) to reduce swelling and prevent movement of the injured hand.

SUPPORT hand and arm in elevation sling

TIE binder bandage around arm and body

3 Tie a BINDER BANDAGE (see p.76 and 80) around the arm, securing it with a knot tied on the uninjured side.
✛ TAKE YOUR CHILD TO THE HOSPITAL

83

TRAPPED FINGERS

COOL injury by holding her fingers under running water

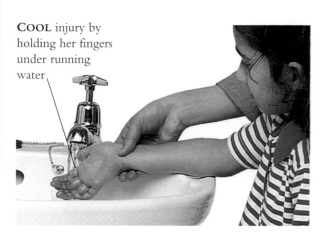

After the trapped fingers are released, hold them under cold running water for a few minutes to relieve the pain and minimize swelling. If the fingers still hurt, apply a COLD COMPRESS (see p.84).

IF *after half an hour the fingers are still swollen and movement is impaired, they may be broken.*
✛ TAKE YOUR CHILD TO THE HOSPITAL

BRUISES AND SWELLINGS

After a fall or bump, bruising and swelling may develop rapidly. Resting, cooling, and elevating the injury will alleviate symptoms.

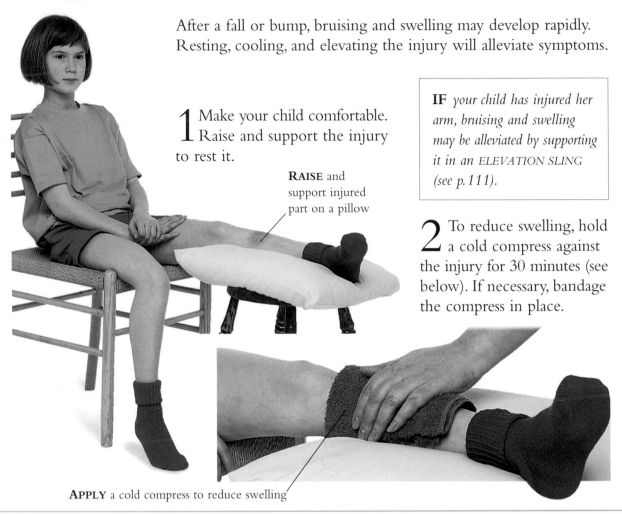

1 Make your child comfortable. Raise and support the injury to rest it.

RAISE and support injured part on a pillow

> **IF** *your child has injured her arm, bruising and swelling may be alleviated by supporting it in an ELEVATION SLING (see p.111).*

2 To reduce swelling, hold a cold compress against the injury for 30 minutes (see below). If necessary, bandage the compress in place.

APPLY a cold compress to reduce swelling

84

Making a cold compress

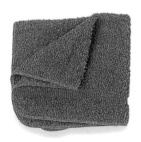

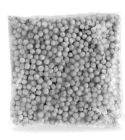

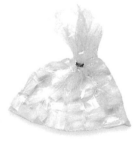

A cold compress minimizes swelling and pain by reducing blood flow to the injured area. Leave a compress on the injury for about 30 minutes, changing it as necessary. If possible, the compress should be left uncovered, but if you need to secure it in place, use a gauze bandage or other open-weave material.

Cloth: wring it out in cold water and replace every ten minutes.

Bag of frozen peas: wrap in a light towel before placing it on the injury.

Ice: fill a plastic bag two-thirds full of ice and add a little salt to help the ice melt, then seal.

SPLINTER

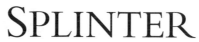

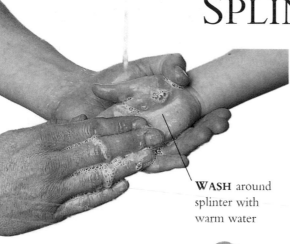

WASH around splinter with warm water

1 Clean the area around the splinter with soap and warm water.

> **IF** *your child is not immunized against TETANUS (p.50),* ℂ CALL A DOCTOR

> **DO NOT** *poke at the area with a needle.*

2 Sterilize a pair of tweezers by passing them through a flame. Let the tweezers cool. Don't touch the ends or wipe off the soot.

STERILIZE tweezers in a flame

85

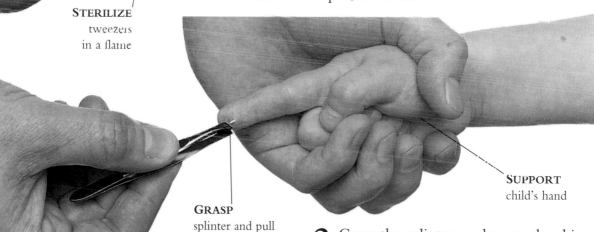

SUPPORT child's hand

GRASP splinter and pull straight out

3 Grasp the splinter as close to the skin as possible, and draw it back out at the angle it went in.

> **IF** *the splinter doesn't come out easily, or if it breaks,* ℂ CALL A DOCTOR

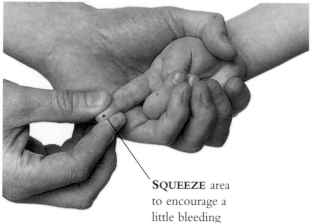

SQUEEZE area to encourage a little bleeding

4 Squeeze the wound gently to encourage a little bleeding that will flush out dirt. Wash the area again, pat it dry thoroughly, and cover with a bandage.

EYE

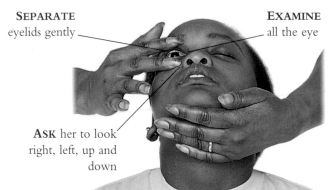

SEPARATE eyelids gently

EXAMINE all the eye

ASK her to look right, left, up and down

> **DO NOT** *touch, or attempt to remove, any foreign object that is sticking to, or embedded in, the eye (see below).*

1 Sit your child down, facing the light. Separate the eyelids. Ask her to look right, left, up, and down. Examine all of the eye.

TRY to wash out foreign object

LIFT off foreign object with a damp hankerchief

USE a bowl to catch water

2 If you can see the foreign object, wash it out using a jug of clean water. Tilt her head and aim for the inner corner so that water will wash over the eye. Or, use the corner of a damp handkerchief to lift it off.

3 If an object is under the eyelid, you can ask an older child to clear it by lifting the upper eyelid over the lower. You will need to do this for a younger child; wrap her in a towel first to stop her from grabbing your arms.

LIFT upper eyelid over lower lid

> **IF** *eye is still red or sore,*
> ✚ TAKE HER TO THE HOSPITAL

A foreign object that cannot be removed

Cover the eye with a protective cover. Do not put pressure on the eye. Reassure him.
✚ TAKE HIM TO THE HOSPITAL
OR ☎ CALL 911

COVER injured eye

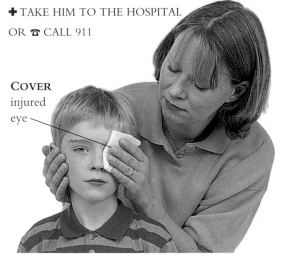

86

EAR

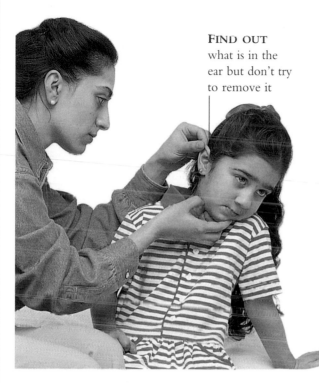

FIND OUT what is in the ear but don't try to remove it

Children often push things into their ears. A hard object may become stuck, causing pain and temporary deafness; it may damage the ear drum.

> **DO NOT** *attempt to remove the object.*

Reassure your child and ask her what she put into her ear. Don't try to remove the object, even if you can see it.

✚ TAKE YOUR CHILD TO THE HOSPITAL.

An insect in the ear

If an insect flies or crawls into the ear your child may be very alarmed. Sit her down and support her head with the affected ear uppermost. Gently flood the ear with lukewarm water so that the insect floats out.

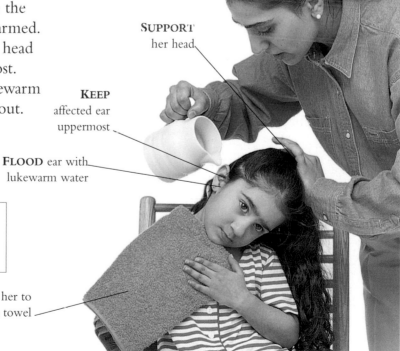

SUPPORT her head

KEEP affected ear uppermost

FLOOD ear with lukewarm water

ASK her to hold a towel

> **IF** *you can't remove the insect,*
> ✚ TAKE YOUR CHILD TO THE HOSPITAL

NOSE

Recognizing a foreign object in the nose
• *Difficult or noisy breathing through nose* • *Swelling of nose* • *Smelly or blood-stained discharge indicates object has been present for a while*

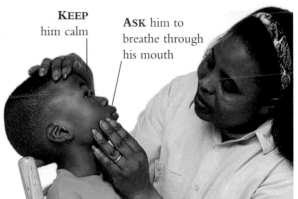

KEEP him calm

ASK him to breathe through his mouth

Calm and reassure your child and tell him to breathe through his mouth.

> **DO NOT** *attempt to remove the object.*
> ✚ TAKE YOUR CHILD TO THE HOSPITAL

SWALLOWED OBJECT

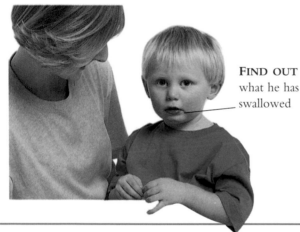

FIND OUT what he has swallowed

Find out what your child has swallowed. If the object is small and smooth like a pebble or a coin, there is little danger.

𝒞 CALL A DOCTOR

> **IF** *the object is sharp or large, or if your child has pain with swallowing or is drooling, don't give your child anything to eat or drink.*
> ✚ TAKE YOUR CHILD TO THE HOSPITAL

INHALED FOREIGN OBJECT

Small, smooth objects can slip into the air passages. Peanuts are a danger in young children as they can be inhaled into the lungs.

Your child will cough violently and this may expel the object. If he continues to choke, see CHOKING BABY, p.36; CHOKING CHILD, p.38.

𝒞 CALL A DOCTOR
OR
☎ CALL 911

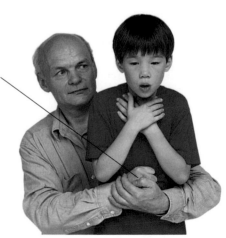

GIVE abdominal thrusts if he continues to choke

ANIMAL BITE
Superficial bite

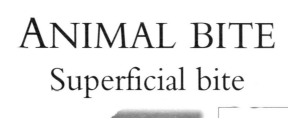

> **MAKE** *sure he is protected against tetanus infection (see p.50).*

WASH wound with soap and warm, running water

1 Wash the wound thoroughly, using soap and warm water. Rinse the wound under running water for at least five minutes to wash away any dirt.

2 Gently, but thoroughly, pat the wound dry with a clean pad or tissue. Cover it with a bandage or a small sterile dressing.

DRY wound and cover with a bandage

🕐 CALL A DOCTOR

Serious bite

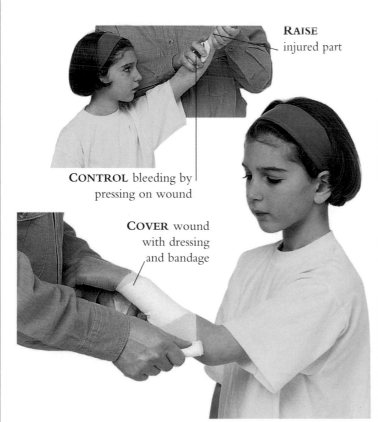

RAISE injured part

CONTROL bleeding by pressing on wound

COVER wound with dressing and bandage

1 Apply direct pressure over the wound, preferably over a clean dressing or pad. Lift and support the injured part above the level of your child's heart.

> **IF** *the bleeding is severe, see* BLEEDING, *p.46.*

2 Cover the wound with a sterile dressing or pad and bandage firmly in place.
+ TAKE YOUR CHILD TO THE HOSPITAL

> **REPORT** *the bite to the police or other agency. If the animal is unknown or cannot be found, it may be necessary to immunize your child against rabies.*

89

INSECT STING

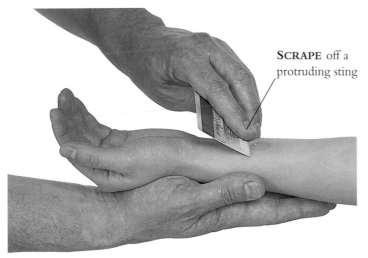

SCRAPE off a protruding sting

1 If the sting is still in the skin, brush or scrape it off sideways. Do not try to remove it with tweezers as you will inject more poison into your child.

> **IF** *your child collapses, she may be allergic to the sting. Follow the treatment for ANAPHYLACTIC SHOCK, opposite.*

Sting in mouth

To reduce swelling, give your child an ice cube to suck or cold water to drink.

✆ CALL A DOCTOR

IF her breathing becomes difficult, ☎ CALL 911

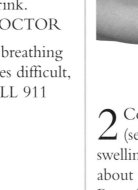

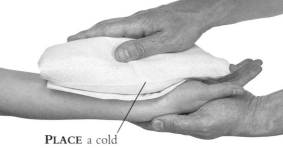

PLACE a cold compress over area

2 Cool the area with a COLD COMPRESS (see p.84) to minimize the pain and swelling. Leave the compress in place for about ten minutes, until the pain is relieved. Rest the injured part.

HIVES

To relieve the itching, dab the rash with cotton soaked in calamine lotion. Alternatively, place a COLD COMPRESS (see p.84) over the rash until the pain is relieved, about ten minutes. If the rash is extensive,

✆ CALL A DOCTOR

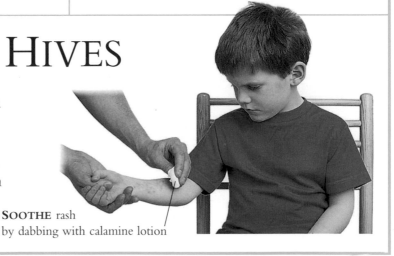

SOOTHE rash by dabbing with calamine lotion

ANAPHYLACTIC SHOCK

This is a severe allergic reaction that may develop within a few minutes following the injection of a particular drug, the sting of an insect or marine creature, or the ingestion of a particular food. Anaphylactic shock by definition implies that at least two body systems are involved. One of these is always the respiratory tract. The other system can vary, but might be the skin.

The reaction causes constriction of the air passages. Swelling of the face and neck increases the risk of suffocation.

Recognizing anaphylactic shock
- *Anxiety* • *Red, blotchy skin* • *Swelling of the face and neck* • *Puffiness around the eyes*
- *Wheezing* • *Difficult breathing* • *Rapid pulse*

☎ CALL 911 IMMEDIATELY

If your child loses consciousness, assess his condition (see UNCONSCIOUS BABY, p. 16; UNCONSCIOUS CHILD, p. 22). If breathing, place him in the recovery position (p. 24). Be prepared to resuscitate.

A CHILD *with a known allergy may have medication to take in case of an attack. This medication usually takes the form of a syringe or autoinjector of epinephrine ("Epipen") prescribed for the child's own use. Help the child use the medication or, if trained, give it yourself. Follow the directions carefully.*

Help your child into the position that most relieves his breathing difficulty. Talk to him calmly and reassure him while you wait for the ambulance to arrive.

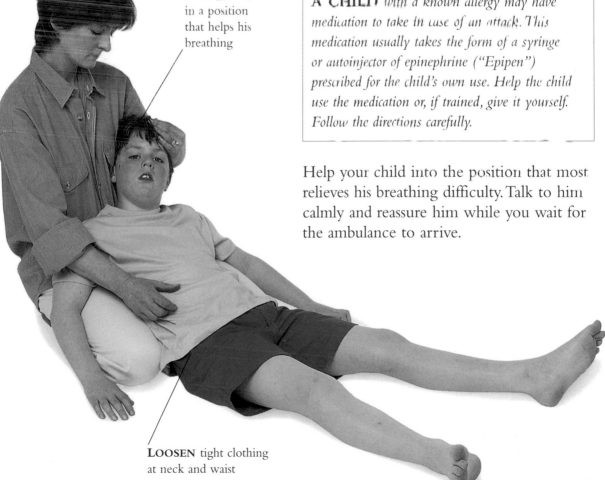

SUPPORT him in a position that helps his breathing

LOOSEN tight clothing at neck and waist

91

MARINE STINGS
Jellyfish sting

Jellyfish venom is contained in stinging cells that stick to a child's skin. The sting is painful, but not usually serious. A similar reaction is produced by sea anemones and corals.

IF *your child develops a severe allergic reaction, see* ANAPHYLACTIC SHOCK, *p.91.* ☎ CALL 911

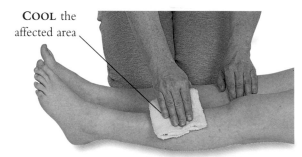

COOL the affected area

1 Apply a cold compress against the skin for about ten minutes.

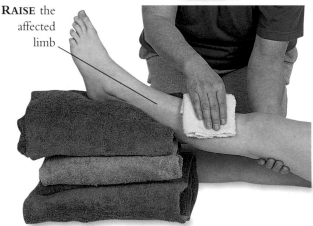

RAISE the affected limb

2 If possible, raise the affected part to reduce swelling.

IF *the skin is very red and painful,*
✚TAKE YOUR CHILD TO THE HOSPITAL

Marine puncture wounds

When stepped on, the spines from sea urchins and some species of fish can puncture the skin, causing painful swelling and soreness. The spines may break off and become embedded in the foot.

Immerse the injury in hot water for at least 30 minutes. Add more hot water as the water cools down.

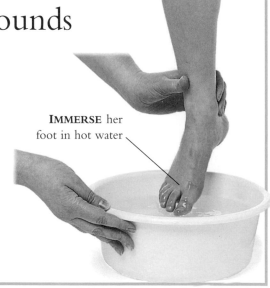

IMMERSE her foot in hot water

IF *any spines remain, or the foot starts to swell,*
✚TAKE YOUR CHILD TO THE HOSPITAL

92

SNAKE BITE

Recognizing a snake bite • *A pair of puncture marks* • *Severe pain, redness, and swelling around bite* • *Vomiting* • *Disturbed vision* • *Breathing difficulties* • *Increased salivation and sweating*

IF *your child develops* ANAPHYLACTIC SHOCK, *see p.91.* **IF** *he loses consciousness, see* UNCONSCIOUS BABY, *p.16;* UNCONSCIOUS CHILD, *p.22. Be prepared to resuscitate. If breathing, place him in the* RECOVERY POSITION *(see p.24).*

DO NOT *let your child walk.*
DO NOT *apply a tourniquet, cut out the wound, or try to suck out the venom.*
An accurate description of the snake will help doctors treat the injury.

1 Make sure area is safe. Help your child lie down. Keep the heart above the level of the bite area to contain the poison.

2 Gently wash the wound and pat dry with clean swabs.

CLEAN and dry the wound

93

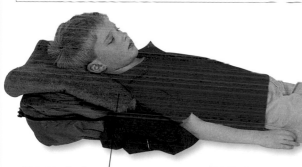

RAISE the heart above the level of the bite

APPLY a gauze wrap bandage above the wound

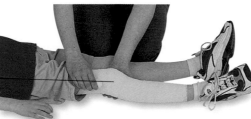

3 Lightly compress the limb above the wound with a gauze wrap bandage. If the hand or foot begins to feel numb or cold, loosen the bandages slightly.

4 Immobilize the limb with folded triangular bandages and padding.

5 Reassure him. Keep him still to stop the venom from spreading through his body.

☎ CALL 911

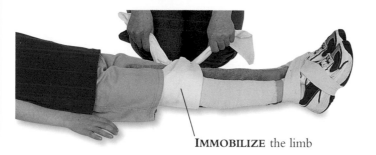

IMMOBILIZE the limb

HYPOTHERMIA

Hypothermia occurs when the body temperature falls. Deep hypothermia, where the body temperature has fallen to a very low level, is extremely dangerous. An older child is most likely to develop hypothermia after overexertion outside in poor weather conditions, or after falling into very cold water. For babies, see opposite.

GIVE her a warm bath

Recognizing hypothermia
• *Shivering* • *Cold, pale, dry skin*
• *Listlessness or confusion* • *Decreasing consciousness* • *Slow, shallow breathing*
• *Weakening pulse*

1 Give your child a warm bath, if she is able to climb in herself. When her skin color has returned to normal, help her out, dry her quickly, and wrap her in warm towels or blankets.

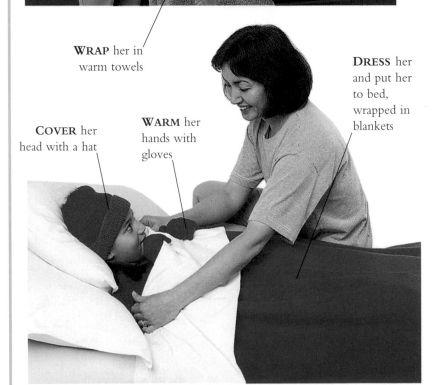

WRAP her in warm towels

DRESS her and put her to bed, wrapped in blankets

COVER her head with a hat

WARM her hands with gloves

2 Dress your child with warm clothes and put her to bed, covered with plenty of blankets. Cover her head with a hat and make sure that the room is warm. Stay with her.

✆ CALL A DOCTOR

DO NOT *put a source of direct heat, such as a hot-water bottle, next to the child's skin. The child must warm up gradually.*

94

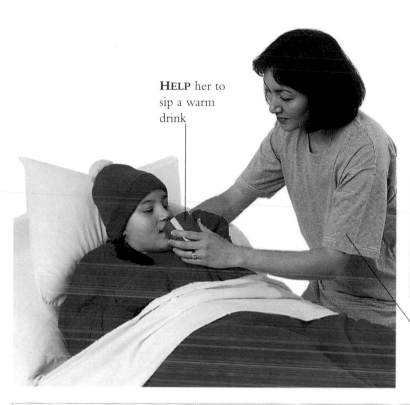

HELP her to sip a warm drink

3 Give your child a warm drink and some high-calorie foods, such as chocolate. Do not leave her alone until you are sure that her color and temperature have returned to normal.

> **IF** *your child loses consciousness, assess her condition (see* UNCONSCIOUS BABY p.16; UNCONSCIOUS CHILD p.22). *Be prepared to resuscitate.*
> ☎ CALL 911

STAY with her until color and temperature have returned to normal

Hypothermia in babies

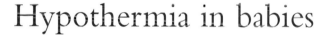

A baby's temperature regulation is not fully developed. He may lose body warmth rapidly and develop hypothermia in a cold room. A hypothermic baby must be warmed gradually.
Recognizing hypothermia in babies • *Pink and healthy-looking skin that feels cold* • *Baby seems limp and unusually quiet* • *Refuses to feed*

☎ CALL 911

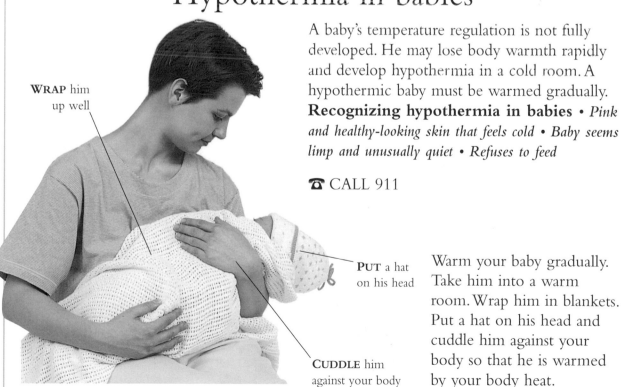

WRAP him up well

PUT a hat on his head

CUDDLE him against your body

Warm your baby gradually. Take him into a warm room. Wrap him in blankets. Put a hat on his head and cuddle him against your body so that he is warmed by your body heat.

FROSTBITE

If children are accidentally exposed to extremely cold weather conditions, the tissues of the fingers and toes may freeze. Get your child to shelter before you start treatment.

Recognizing frostbite • *Pins and needles* • *Numbing* • *Skin feeling hard and stiff, turning white, and waxy*

REMOVE clothing from affected area carefully

TAKE her gloves off very carefully

96

1 Take your child into a warm place. Sit her down then very gently remove her socks and shoes.

2 Remove gloves and any rings. Undo her coat. Tell her to warm her hands under her armpits.

WARM hands with her own body heat, under armpits

3 When the feet or toes are frozen, to reduce swelling and provide warmth, raise your child's feet and warm her toes under your own armpits.

USE your body heat to thaw feet

DO NOT *warm by rubbing or with direct heat, such as hot-water bottles.* **NEVER** *burst blisters.*

COVER with light dressing and bandage if color does not return

4 If the skin is broken or the color does not return rapidly, apply a soft gauze dressing and bandage it lightly in place.
✚ TAKE YOUR CHILD TO THE HOSPITAL

HEAT EXHAUSTION

This condition may develop in hot, humid weather and is caused by dehydration. Children who are unwell, particularly with diarrhea and vomiting, and those not used to playing in the heat are most at risk.

Recognizing heat exhaustion • *Headache and dizziness* • *Nausea* • *Sweating* • *Pale, clammy skin* • *Cramps* • *Rapid, weakening pulse*

1 Take your child into the shade or into a cool room. Help him to lie down.

LAY child down in cool room

PUT folded towel or cushion under his head

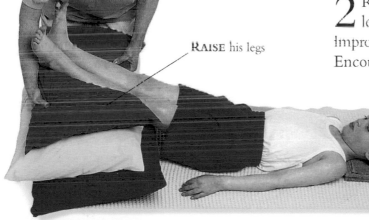

RAISE his legs

2 Raise and support your child's legs on some pillows. This improves blood supply to the brain. Encourage him to rest.

97

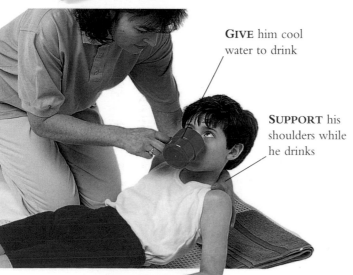

GIVE him cool water to drink

SUPPORT his shoulders while he drinks

3 Help your child to sit up and sip as much cool water or juice as he can manage. This replaces fluid lost from the body.

IF *he loses consciousness, assess his condition (see* UNCONSCIOUS BABY *p16;* UNCONSCIOUS CHILD, *p.22). Be prepared to resuscitate. If breathing, place him in the* RECOVERY POSITION *(see p.24).*
☎ CALL 911

HEATSTROKE

If the body becomes severely overheated in hot surroundings, heatstroke may occur.

Recognizing heatstroke

- *Sudden onset of headache*
- *Sweating stops • Confusion*
- *Hot, flushed, dry skin*
- *Rapid deterioration in level of response • A full, bounding pulse • Temperature above 104°F (40°C)*

IF *a baby or young child develops heatstroke, undress him completely and sponge him down (see p.101).*
☎ CALL 911

☎ **CALL 911**

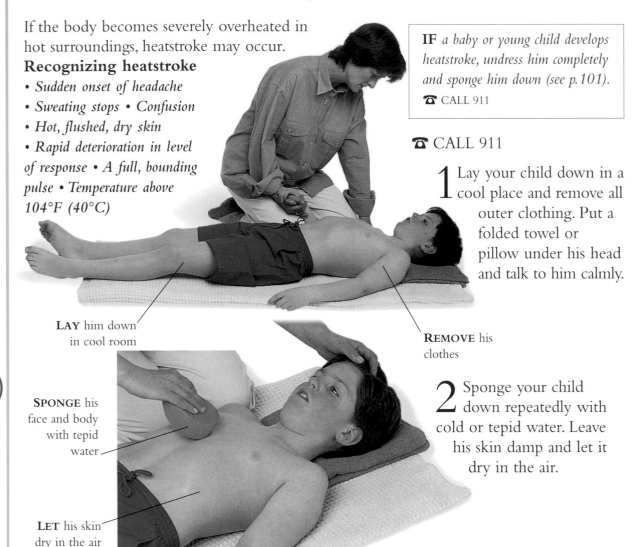

1 Lay your child down in a cool place and remove all outer clothing. Put a folded towel or pillow under his head and talk to him calmly.

LAY him down in cool room

REMOVE his clothes

SPONGE his face and body with tepid water

2 Sponge your child down repeatedly with cold or tepid water. Leave his skin damp and let it dry in the air.

LET his skin dry in the air

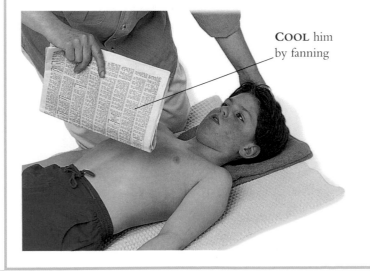

COOL him by fanning

3 Fan your child by hand or with an electric fan to bring his temperature down.

IF *he loses consciousness, assess his condition (see UNCONSCIOUS BABY, p.16; UNCONSCIOUS CHILD, p.22). Be prepared to resuscitate. If breathing, place him in the RECOVERY POSITION (see p.24).*
☎ CALL 911

98

SUNBURN

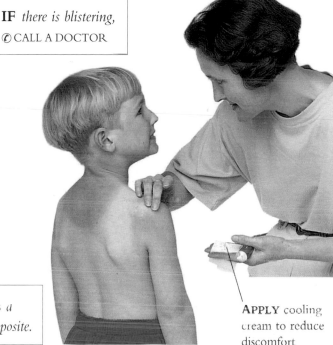

TAKE him into shade

GIVE him cold water to sip

Sunburn is red, itchy, and tender. Babies and young children are particularly vulnerable and should wear a hat and protective cream or clothing in the sun.

> **IF** *there is blistering,*
> Ⓒ CALL A DOCTOR

1 Move your child into the shade or into a cool room and give him a cold drink.

2 Apply calamine cream or a special after-sun cream to soothe the skin.

> **IF** *your child is restless, flushed, dizzy, or has a temperature or headache, see* HEATSTROKE, *opposite.*

APPLY cooling cream to reduce discomfort

99

HEAT RASH

Recognizing heat rash • *A prickly, red rash particularly around the sweat glands on the chest and back and under the arms*

Sit your child down in a cool room and undress her. Sponge her down with cool water. Pat her almost dry with a soft towel, leaving the skin slightly damp. Apply calamine cream.

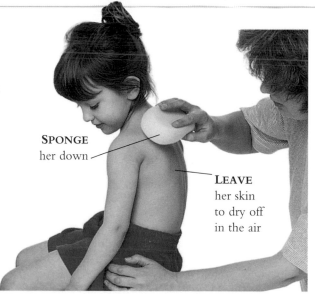

SPONGE her down

LEAVE her skin to dry off in the air

> **IF** *your baby develops heat rash, remove some of her clothes to cool her, or bathe her in tepid water. Dry her gently, leaving her skin slightly damp.*

> **IF** *the rash resembles blood under the skin,*
> ☎ CALL 911

FEVER

A body temperature that is above the normal level of 98.6°F (37°C) indicates fever. An infection is the usual cause. If your child also has a bad headache, you should study the information on MENINGITIS (see opposite). A moderate fever is not harmful, but a temperature of above 104°F (40°C) can indicate serious illness, especially in babies and very young children. Any infant under three months old with a temperature higher than 100°F (38°C) should see a doctor immediately.

Recognizing a fever • *Raised temperature* • *A very pale face and a chilled feeling, with goose pimples* • *Shivering, with chattering teeth* As the fever advances • *Hot, flushed skin* • *General achiness* • *Sweating* • *Headache*

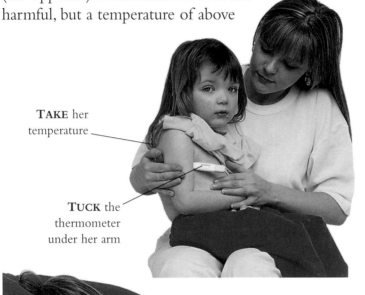

TAKE her temperature

TUCK the thermometer under her arm

LAY her down in bed or on the sofa

PROVIDE her with plenty to drink

GIVE her recommended dose of liquid acetaminophen

1 Lift your child's arm and tuck the pointed end of the thermometer into her armpit. Fold her arm over her chest and leave the thermometer in place for the recommended time. A digital thermometer is the easiest to use.

2 Make your child comfortable on a bed or sofa, but do not cover her. To help bring down her temperature, make sure she has plenty of water or diluted fruit juice to drink.

3 You can give your child the recommended dose of liquid acetaminophen for her weight to help reduce her temperature (see opposite).

> **IF** *your baby is under three months old, she should not be given liquid acetaminophen, unless you are advised to do so by your doctor.*
> Ⓒ CALL A DOCTOR

100

Cooling babies and young children

In babies and children under five years of age, there is some risk of FEBRILE SEIZURES (see p.32). This is often familial and happens with rapid rise in temperature. ⓒ CALL A DOCTOR.

Undress your child (or your baby down to her diaper) and cool her by giving the weight-appropriate dose of acetaminophen every four hours. Try to keep her calm. A baby under three months old should see a doctor immediately. If sponging is recommended by your doctor, ensure that the sponge is just damp, not too wet, and the water is tepid, not cold.

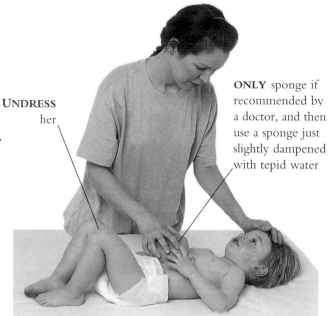

UNDRESS her

ONLY sponge if recommended by a doctor, and then use a sponge just slightly dampened with tepid water

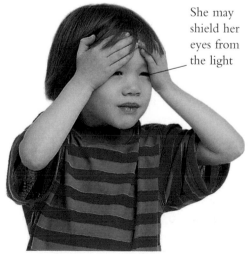

SPONGE only if recommended by a doctor

> **FEVER** *can also be caused by too much sun, see* HEATSTROKE, *p.98.*

Meningitis

She may shield her eyes from the light

This is a serious condition involving the tissues that surround the brain. It is frequently life-threatening and urgent treatment is essential.

Recognizing meningitis • *Fever* • *Vomiting* • *Headache* • *Neck pain or stiff neck* • *Seizures* • *A red or purple rash that does not fade when pressure is applied* • *Pain in the eyes caused by light* • *Child unable to bend her neck to touch her chin to her chest*

ⓒ CALL A DOCTOR IMMEDIATELY
IF *there is any delay in help arriving,* ✚ TAKE YOUR CHILD TO THE HOSPITAL OR ☎ CALL 911

VOMITING

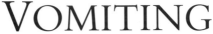

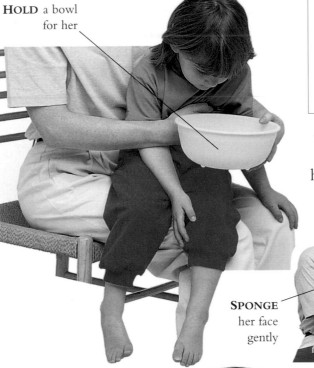

HOLD a bowl
for her

> **A BABY** *suffering repeated vomiting and diarrhea can become dehydrated. Prolonged vomiting may need to be treated with oral rehydration drinks.*
> ⓒ CALL A DOCTOR

1 Hold your child over a bowl or basin. Support her upper body with your free hand while she is vomiting. Reassure her.

2 Once she has stopped vomiting, wipe her face and around her mouth with a sponge or cloth wrung out in tepid water.

SPONGE
her face
gently

102

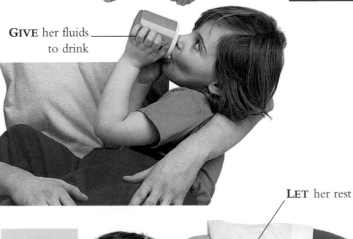

GIVE her fluids
to drink

3 Give her fluids, such as oral rehydration solutions, to replace any fluid loss and to remove the unpleasant taste. Encourage her to sip each drink slowly.

4 Let her rest quietly, in bed if she wants to. Make sure the bowl is still within reach in case of further vomiting, and provide fresh clear fluids.

LET her rest

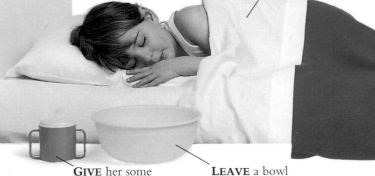

5 To monitor her hydration, check that she is alert and oriented, is passing urine regularly, has tears in her eyes, and a moist tongue.

GIVE her some
fresh fluids

LEAVE a bowl
for her

STOMACHACHE

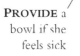

PROP her up against cushions or pillows

1 Make your child comfortable on a sofa or bed. If she is having difficulty breathing, help her to lie back against cushions or pillows. She may want to vomit, so leave a container nearby.

> **IF** *the pain is severe or does not subside after 30 minutes, or if there are breathing problems*
> ℂ CALL A DOCTOR

2 Warmth may help to relieve the pain. Fill a covered hot-water bottle with warm water and give it to your child to hold against her stomach. Do not give her anything to eat and only clear fluids to drink.

PROVIDE a bowl if she feels sick

GIVE her a covered hot-water bottle to hold against her stomach

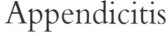

(103)

Appendicitis

Inflammation of the appendix may occur at any age.

Recognizing appendicitis • *Waves of crampy pain in the middle of the abdomen* • *Then acute pain settling in the right lower abdomen* • *Raised temperature* • *Loss of appetite* • *Nausea* • *Vomiting* • *Diarrhea*

> **APPENDICITIS** *must be treated promptly. Help your child lie down on a sofa or bed. Do not give him anything to eat or drink.*
> ℂ CALL A DOCTOR OR ✚ TAKE YOUR CHILD TO THE HOSPITAL

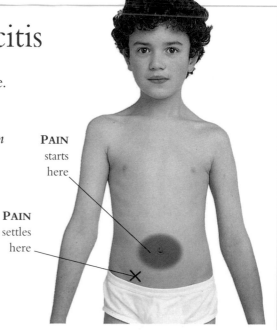

PAIN starts here

PAIN settles here

EARACHE

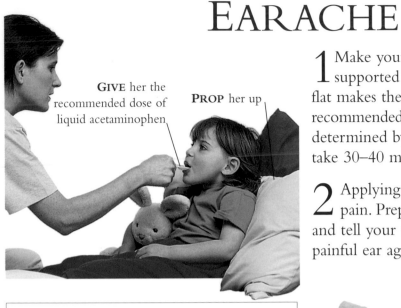

GIVE her the recommended dose of liquid acetaminophen

PROP her up

1 Make your child comfortable. Sit her up supported by pillows or cushions if lying flat makes the earache worse. Give her the recommended dose of liquid acetaminophen, determined by her body weight. This will take 30–40 minutes to take effect.

2 Applying heat may help to soothe the pain. Prepare a covered hot-water bottle and tell your child to lie down with her painful ear against it.

PROVIDE a covered hot-water bottle to place against her ear

IF *pain does not begin to subside, or if there is a discharge from the ear, fever, or hearing loss,* © CALL A DOCTOR

104

Pressure-change earache

This may happen on plane rides, particularly when taking off or landing, or when traveling through tunnels. To make the ears "pop" so that the pressure is relieved, your child should close her mouth, hold her nose, and blow. Sucking a piece of hard candy may also help. Allow babies to suck a bottle or pacifier.

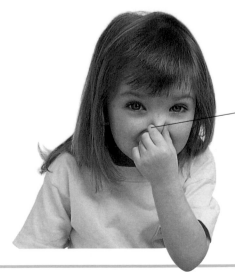

TELL her to pinch her nose, close her mouth, and "blow" her nose

TOOTHACHE

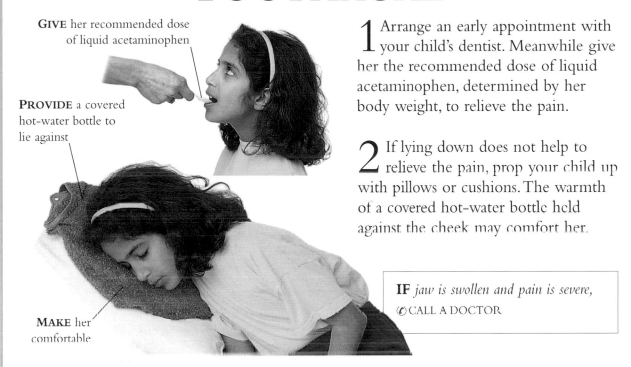

GIVE her recommended dose of liquid acetaminophen

PROVIDE a covered hot-water bottle to lie against

MAKE her comfortable

1 Arrange an early appointment with your child's dentist. Meanwhile give her the recommended dose of liquid acetaminophen, determined by her body weight, to relieve the pain.

2 If lying down does not help to relieve the pain, prop your child up with pillows or cushions. The warmth of a covered hot-water bottle held against the cheek may comfort her.

IF *jaw is swollen and pain is severe,* (☉)CALL A DOCTOR

CRAMP

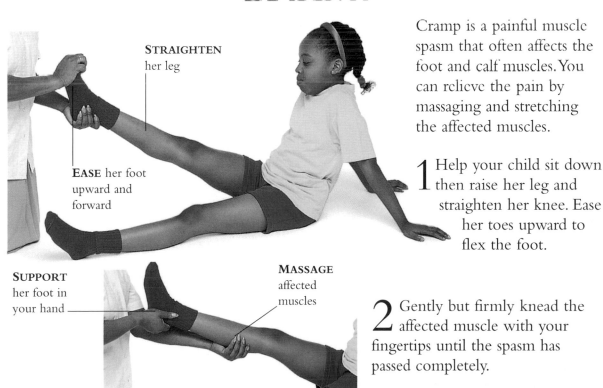

STRAIGHTEN her leg

EASE her foot upward and forward

SUPPORT her foot in your hand

MASSAGE affected muscles

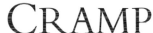

Cramp is a painful muscle spasm that often affects the foot and calf muscles. You can relieve the pain by massaging and stretching the affected muscles.

1 Help your child sit down then raise her leg and straighten her knee. Ease her toes upward to flex the foot.

2 Gently but firmly knead the affected muscle with your fingertips until the spasm has passed completely.

FIRST AID KIT

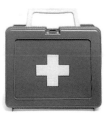

A well-stocked first aid kit
1 small gauze roll
1 large gauze roll
1 small and 1 large elastic bandage
Scissors
Calamine cream
Pack of gauze swabs
2 triangular bandages
Hypoallergenic tape
2 sterile pads
Waterproof adhesive bandages
1 finger bandage and applicator
Tweezers
1 sterile dressing with bandage
Antibiotic ointment

Keep first aid kits in your car and in your home. You can buy ready-made-up standard kits. You may want to add extra dressings and bandages, and disposable gloves. Make sure your first aid box is readily accessible and easy to identify, and check the contents regularly. Don't keep medicines in the first aid box; they should be locked in a medicine cabinet. A well-stocked kit might contain the articles shown below.

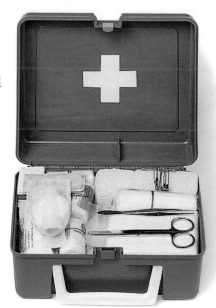

Dressings

Adhesive bandages are used for minor wounds. Keep several different sizes and shapes. Keep a selection of larger sterile dressings for more serious wounds.

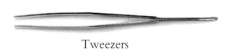

Scissors

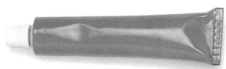

Tweezers

Calamine cream or lotion

Adhesive bandages

Gauze swabs

Sterile nonadhesive pad

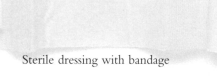

Sterile dressing with bandage

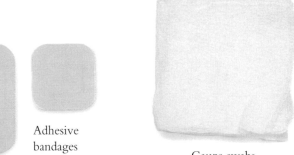

Bandages

Keep a variety of bandages to secure dressings and support injured joints. Gauze rolls are easy to use because they shape themselves to the contours of the body. Triangular bandages can be used as slings and for binder and cravat bandages.

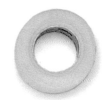

Hypoallergenic tape for securing dressings

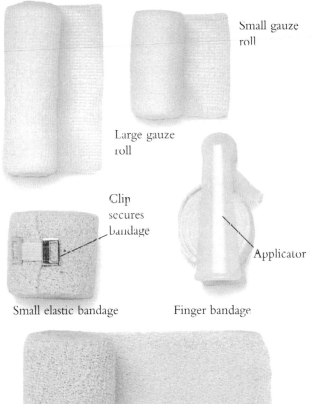

Small gauze roll

Large gauze roll

Clip secures bandage

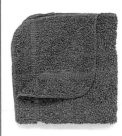

Applicator

Small elastic bandage

Finger bandage

Large elastic bandage

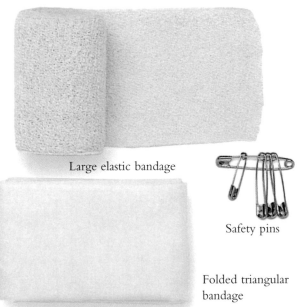

Safety pins

Folded triangular bandage

Other useful items

A variety of household items are invaluable for first aid emergencies. If you don't have exactly the right materials, you can improvise successfully. Keep the following articles to hand.

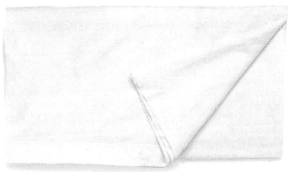

Washcloth

Use a washcloth soaked in water to make a cold compress.

Sheet and pillowcase

A clean cotton sheet or pillowcase makes an excellent loose protective covering for burns.

Plastic wrap

Plastic wrap can be used to seal chest wounds.

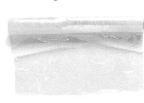

Plastic bags

A clean plastic bag can be put over a burned foot or hand and lightly secured with bandages or tape.

DRESSINGS

Adhesive bandage

Covering a wound with a dressing will help prevent infection and help the blood-clotting process. Dressings should not be fluffy and need to be large enough to cover the wound and the surrounding area. Always wash your hands before you apply dressings and wear disposable gloves if you have them. If blood soaks through a dressing, replace it. Make sure any bandages are not too tight (see opposite).

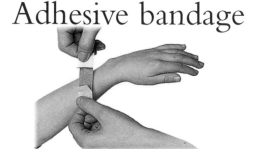

Remove wrapping and, holding the pad over the wound, peel back the protective strips. Press the ends and edges down.

Sterile pad

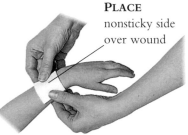

PLACE nonsticky side over wound

BANDAGE the pad in place

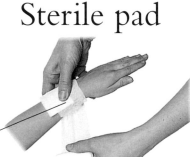

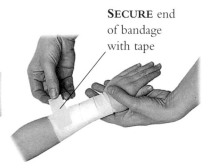

SECURE end of bandage with tape

1 Place the pad shiny side down directly over the wound.

2 Secure the pad with a bandage, working from below the injury up the limb.

3 Secure the end of the bandage with hypoallergenic tape.

Sterile dressing with bandage

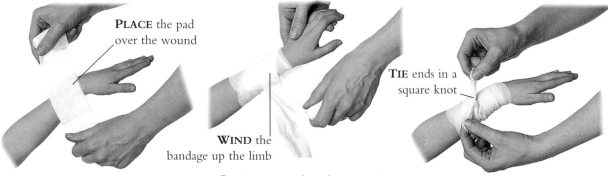

PLACE the pad over the wound

WIND the bandage up the limb

TIE ends in a square knot

1 Hold the bandage either side of the dressing, and place the pad over the wound.

2 Leaving the short end hanging, wind the other end around the limb until the dressing is covered.

3 Tie the two ends of the bandage in a SQUARE KNOT (see p.76), over the pad.

108

BANDAGING

Use bandages to secure dressings, help control bleeding, and to support injuries. Gauze rolls can be used for any part of the body; they are especially useful for bandaging joints or heads because they mold themselves to the shape of the body.

> **DO NOT** *apply a bandage too tightly – it will impair the circulation. To check, press on your child's nail or a patch of skin, then release pressure. The color should return rapidly. If it does not, loosen the bandages.*

Gauze roll

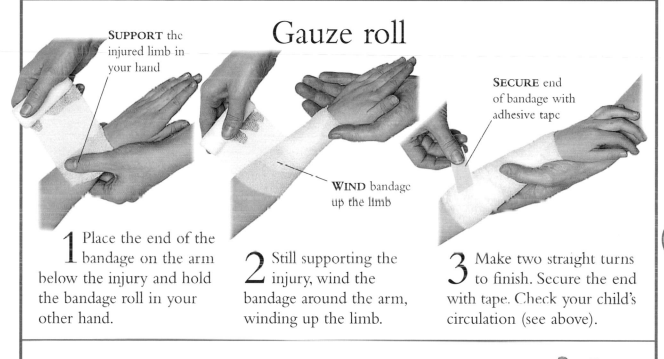

SUPPORT the injured limb in your hand

WIND bandage up the limb

SECURE end of bandage with adhesive tape

1 Place the end of the bandage on the arm below the injury and hold the bandage roll in your other hand.

2 Still supporting the injury, wind the bandage around the arm, winding up the limb.

3 Make two straight turns to finish. Secure the end with tape. Check your child's circulation (see above).

109

Hand bandage

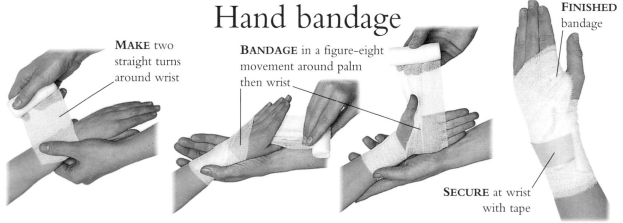

MAKE two straight turns around wrist

BANDAGE in a figure-eight movement around palm then wrist

FINISHED bandage

SECURE at wrist with tape

1 Supporting the injury, hold the end of the bandage on the wrist and make two straight turns.

2 Take the bandage across the back of the hand to the base of the little finger, then around the palm, and up between the thumb and forefinger, and across the back of the hand to the wrist. Repeat the "figure-eight" until the hand is covered.

TRIANGULAR BANDAGES

These are sold singly in sterile packs or can be made from a square of strong fabric folded diagonally in half. Triangular bandages are used for BINDER and CRAVAT BANDAGES (see p.76) or slings. Arm slings support injured arms or wrists, or take weight off an injured shoulder. Elevation slings are used for arm and upper body injuries where bleeding, pain, or swelling need to be reduced. (For SQUARE KNOT, see p.76.)

Arm sling

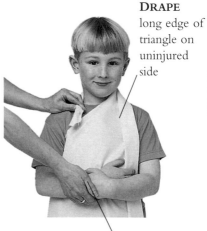

DRAPE long edge of triangle on uninjured side

SUPPORT arm

1 Place the bandage between your child's arm and chest, easing one end up around the back of his neck on the injured side.

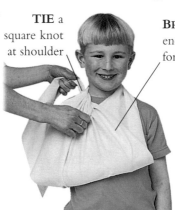

TIE a square knot at shoulder

2 Take the lower end of the bandage over your child's forearm to the end at the shoulder and tie a SQUARE KNOT (see p.76) just below the shoulder.

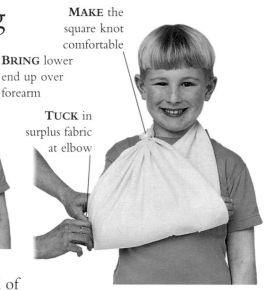

MAKE the square knot comfortable

BRING lower end up over forearm

TUCK in surplus fabric at elbow

3 Fold in the surplus fabric at the corner near the elbow and pin it to the bandage.

Improvised slings

If your child injures her shoulder, arm, or hand out of doors, you can improvise a sling to support the injury until she receives further treatment.

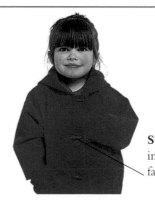

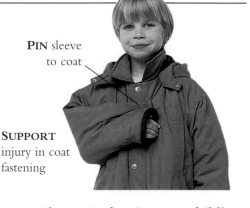

PIN sleeve to coat

SUPPORT injury in coat fastening

Undo a coat button and tuck the hand of the injured arm inside the fastening.

Alternatively, pin your child's sleeve up on the opposite side of his chest.

110

Elevation sling

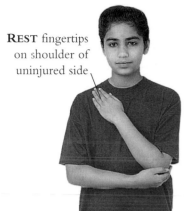

REST fingertips on shoulder of uninjured side

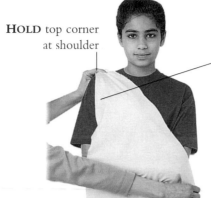

HOLD top corner at shoulder

DRAPE long edge across body

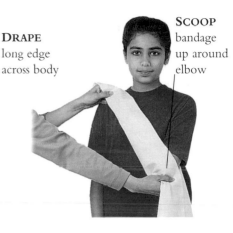

SCOOP bandage up around elbow

1 Bring the arm on the injured side across your child's chest. Ask her to support her elbow.

2 Lay the bandage over your child's arm, with the long edge hanging on the uninjured side. Hold the top corner at the shoulder.

3 Fold long edge of bandage in under injured arm.

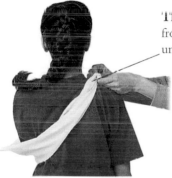

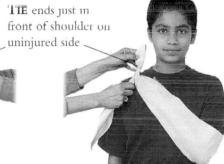

TIE ends just in front of shoulder on uninjured side

4 Bring the other end up around her back, holding the elbow securely in the fabric. Tie a SQUARE KNOT (p.76) just below the shoulder and tuck the ends in.

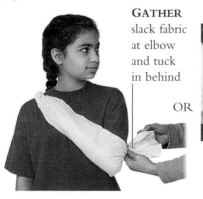

GATHER slack fabric at elbow and tuck in behind

OR

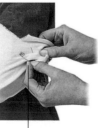

PIN slack fabric to front of sling

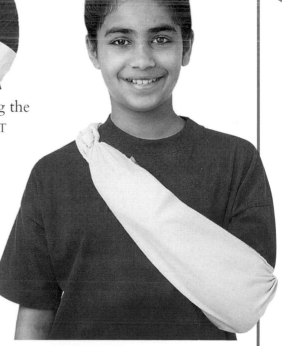

5 Secure the bandage by twisting the excess fabric and tucking it in at the elbow. Pin in place.

Finished sling raises, immobilizes, and supports the injury.

SAFETY IN THE HOME

Most accidents occur at home and over half involve children under the age of five. Many accidents are preventable if you:

- Alter the layout and position of objects and furniture at home.
- Make sure windows are closed or inaccessible.
- Never confuse containers by putting a dangerous substance, such as bleach, in a bottle that used to contain a harmless drink.
- Never tell your child that medicines and pills are special candies.
- Check for potential hazards when visiting friends or relatives and ask if you can move sharp or breakable objects.
- Teach your child basic safety rules.

ELECTRICITY

Protect your child from electric shock (see p.12).

- Cover outlets: put heavy furniture in front of them, or fit plastic covers.
- Put only one or two plugs into each outlet – overloading can start a fire.
- Wire plugs safely – follow instructions and check that you have the right fuse.
- Check that old cords are not worn – a child may try to chew protruding wires.
- Coil cords neatly.
- Fit a GFCI (ground fault circuit interrupter).

112

TEACH your child to recognize hazards

GAS

Find out where your gas valve is in case there is a leak. If you smell gas:

- Don't turn the lights on or off or use any electric switches – there might be a spark, which could cause an explosion.
- Don't light matches or cigarettes.
- Turn off the gas.
- Open the windows.
- Leave the house, then call the gas company.

FIRE

If fire breaks out at home, it could be a matter of minutes before smoke overcomes you.

Fit at least one smoke detector per floor
If your house is on one level, install a detector between the livingroom and the bedrooms. If your house is on two or more levels, install one detector at the foot of the stairs and another outside the bedrooms upstairs.

Have an escape plan (see p. 11). Make sure the whole family knows what to do if there is a fire. Teach older children to "stop, drop, and roll" if their clothes catch fire.

Practice a fire drill with your children

- Shout "fire" • Set off the smoke detector • Tell everyone to drop to the floor and crawl to the exit from the room • Shut the door behind you
- Don't go back for pets or treasured possessions
- Meet outside the house.

> **KEEP** *emergency numbers by the telephone, and make sure everyone knows where they are.*

HALL AND STAIRS

The staircase is not a safe place for your child to play (see below).

- Make sure that toys are not left there for you to trip over.
- Put a light in your hall or on the landing in case your child gets up at night. Use a low-watt bulb, never cover a lamp with a cloth because the cloth can easily catch fire.
- Don't let your child play on the landings or stairs of a communal area in apartment buildings because the banisters may have large gaps between them.

FRONT DOOR

- Don't leave your front door open.
- Don't let your child answer the door for strangers.
- Put the door knob out of reach of small children. If your toddler can reach the knob, fix an additional bolt higher up the door and always keep the door bolted.
- Glass doors should be made with tempered safety glass or laminated glass.
- Put stickers over the glass to make it more noticeable for young children.

FLOOR

Tiled, polished, or sisal-covered floors can be very slippery for toddlers and running children.

- Put nonslip webbing under rugs.
- Keep hall floors free of toys and clutter.
- Check wall-to-wall carpeting regularly for holes or loose carpet that might catch a toddler's foot.

STAIRS

A child is not coordinated enough to be able to walk downstairs safely until he is at least three years old.

- Fit stair gates at the foot and top of the stairs. Vertical posts on stair gates should be no more than 4in (10cm) apart. A young child can get through a larger gap and fall, or get his head stuck. Always open the gate when you are going upstairs or downstairs. Do not climb over it. your children will learn from you.
- Check your banisters for safety. Make sure the handrail is sturdy and check regularly for loose posts. Posts should be no more than 4in (10cm) apart. Do not let your child use the rails as a jungle gym.
- Check the stair carpet. Loose carpet or worn steps can be a hazard.

113

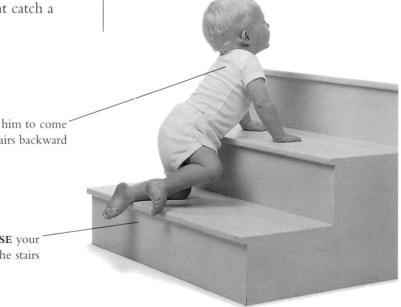

TEACH him to come downstairs backward

SUPERVISE your toddler on the stairs

KITCHEN

The kitchen may be the busiest part of your house, where you spend a lot of time with your children. Constant bustle and cooking activities make it a potentially hazardous area.

DOOR

- Any glass panels should be made of tempered safety glass or laminated glass in case your toddler runs into the door.
- Put some colorful stickers on the glass to alert your child.

FLOOR

- Don't let your child play on the area of floor between you and the work surface or where you could trip over him.
- Avoid bumps and falls by wiping up spills immediately.
- Remove pet food bowls after use and keep that part of the floor scrupulously clean.
- Clean up toys and clutter from underfoot.

TRASH CANS

- Discourage toddlers from rummaging in the garbage and trash cans.
- Put sharp-edged cans and lids or broken glass straight into the trash can.
- Keep the garbage can in a cabinet with a child-resistant safety catch.

> **KEEP** *a fire blanket in the kitchen for smothering flare-ups. If you want to buy a fire extinguisher, consult your local fire department to find out which is the most appropriate type. For more on fires, see p.11 and p.112.*

Babies

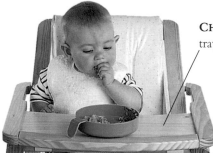

CHECK that removable trays have strong clasps

ATTACH a safety harness to the clips on either side of the chair

HIGHCHAIRS

- Always use a safety harness.
- Never leave the chair where your baby can reach out and pull objects down from a surface. Keep him amused with a safe toy.
- Never leave your child unattended.

BOTTLES AND FOOD

- Wash all your baby's feeding equipment thoroughly.
- Don't leave a prepared meal standing at room temperature, and don't keep the remains of the last meal. Warmed or reheated meals are breeding grounds for bacteria that might upset your baby's stomach.

PLAY

- Have a safe area or a playpen where your baby can play and watch you.
- Keep him out of range of any spills from the stove.

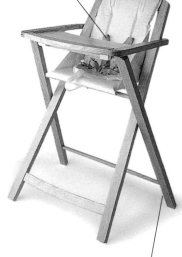

CHOOSE a stable highchair with widely spaced legs.

TABLES AND WORK SURFACES

- Always be aware of your child's reach and keep all heavy, breakable, or sharp objects well back from the edges of tables and work areas.
- Keep stools or chairs away from tables and work surfaces to prevent your child from climbing up on them.
- Tuck cords of kettles, toasters, blenders, and irons out of reach. Choose a curly cord for your kettle if possible. It is not only boiling, steaming kettles that pose a hazard: water is still hot enough to scald 15 minutes after boiling.
- Unplug electrical appliances when not in use.
- Avoid using a tablecloth. It is tempting for a crawling baby or toddler to use it to pull himself up, bringing anything on the table down upon his head. Use place mats instead, or secure the cloth with clips.
- Do not put your baby on a table or work surface when he is in a car seat or bouncing cradle: he could easily fall off.

CABINETS AND DRAWERS

- Put safety catches on cabinets and drawers, particularly those that contain: knives, scissors, and utensils; heavy pots, pans, or china; dried food, such as lentils or pasta, that may be a choking hazard; alcohol and bottles; medicines, including vitamins; cleaning materials, such as laundry soap or bleach, including those with "child-resistant" lids.

REFRIGERATOR

Food poisoning can be caused by poor food storage. Take precautions to minimize risks:

- Keep cooked meat and poultry on a separate shelf from uncooked meat. Cover uncooked meat with plastic wrap.
- Don't store food in open cans; transfer leftovers into a clean container and put in the refrigerator.
- Check food regularly, to see that nothing is kept beyond the "sell-by" date.

STOVE

Your child is obviously at risk of burns and scalds from hot fat or boiling water when you are preparing food.

- You can buy safety guards, but remember that a child can still poke fingers through some types and be burned by hot electric or gas burners.
- Always keep your child away from oven doors; they can get very hot while the oven is in use and will stay hot for some time afterward. A crawling baby or toddler is particularly at risk. Try to teach your child what "hot" means, so that he understands a warning.
- Keep matches well out of reach in a cabinet with a safety catch.

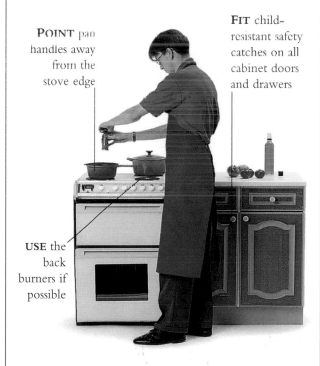

POINT pan handles away from the stove edge

FIT child-resistant safety catches on all cabinet doors and drawers

USE the back burners if possible

WASHING MACHINE AND DRYER

- Keep small hands away from the glass door; it may get hot while the machine is on.
- Ensure that the door is closed while the machine is not in use. Your toddler may try to climb inside or fill it with toys.

LIVING ROOM

While your children are very young, try to arrange the room so that children as well as your valuables are kept out of harm's way. If you have a balcony, block up gaps in the railings with particleboard and check that your child can't climb over. Never leave toys on a high surface because he may attempt to retrieve them.

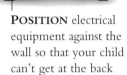

CARPETS AND CURTAINS
- Check that there are no areas of carpet or rug that have holes or turned up edges; either you or your child could trip.
- Wind up and tuck away curtain ties and cords for blinds. Children can be strangled if they get caught in dangling cords.

FIREPLACES AND HEATERS
- Don't leave matches or lighters where your child can reach them.
- Use a firescreen in front of an open fire. Attach it to the wall to prevent your child pulling it over. Put a guard over gas heaters.
- Never use the firescreen as a shelf or clothes dryer.
- Use a spark-guard as well as a firescreen for open fires as an additional precaution.

TELEVISIONS, VIDEOS, AND STEREO EQUIPMENT
- Tack wiring to the baseboard.
- Run long cords behind furniture, so that your child won't trip or pull on them.
- Cover any unused outlets with plastic safety covers.
- Check that old cords are not worn.

POSITION electrical equipment against the wall so that your child can't get at the back

SURFACES AND FURNITURE
- Place houseplants out of reach of young children. Some houseplants are poisonous, and others can scratch or produce allergic reactions if touched.
- Keep breakable or heavy objects off low tables and well back from the edges of surfaces such as window sills or mantelpieces.
- Remove glass-topped tables and put corner protectors on sharp table corners.
- Don't leave hot drinks, alcohol, glasses, cigarettes, matches, or lighters on low surfaces, such as coffee tables, where your child can reach them.
  - Keep alcohol in a locked cabinet.
  - Never leave a cigarette burning on the arm of a sofa or armchair. Old foam furniture can be lethal in a fire because it releases toxic fumes within seconds of catching fire.

ENSURE that bookcases are secured to the wall

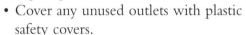

CHOOSE sofas and armchairs with fire-resistant fillings and coverings

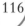

TOYS AND PLAYTHINGS

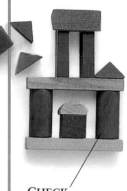

When you buy toys or equipment for your child, follow these guidelines:

- Buy toys that are appropriate for the age of your child and buy from a reputable source.
- Make sure that there are no sharp edges, and avoid anything made of thin, rigid plastic.
- Buy nontoxic paints or crayons.
- Don't buy your child second-hand toys: they may be covered in paint containing lead.
- Avoid novelty toys that are not designed for young children: look out for warnings on the packaging.

CHECK that sets of building blocks don't have small pieces that could be a choking hazard for your child

CARING FOR TOYS

- Check toys regularly and throw away any broken ones.
- Don't mix batteries – change them all at the same time; otherwise, the strong batteries will make the weak ones very hot.
- Keep toys in a toy box. Toys can bring about accidents or injuries by being left on the floor.

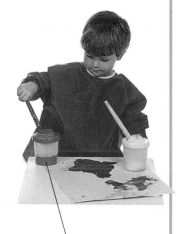

GIVE your child nontoxic paints to play with

117

Babies and toddlers

- Remove ribbons from a baby's soft toys.
- Check that the eyes, noses, ears, or bells on soft toys and dolls are well secured.
- Attach crib toys with a very short string and remove them as soon as your baby can sit up.
- Remove activity centers or bulky toys from a crib as soon as your child can stand, since they provide a foothold for climbing out.
- Don't let babies chew on furry toys: the fur is a choking hazard for children under one year old.
- Never give a small child a toy that is not recommended for his age-group since it may contain small pieces on which he could choke.
- Always supervise a baby or toddler while he is playing.
- Do not use baby walkers.

MAKE SURE that toys that increase mobility are stable

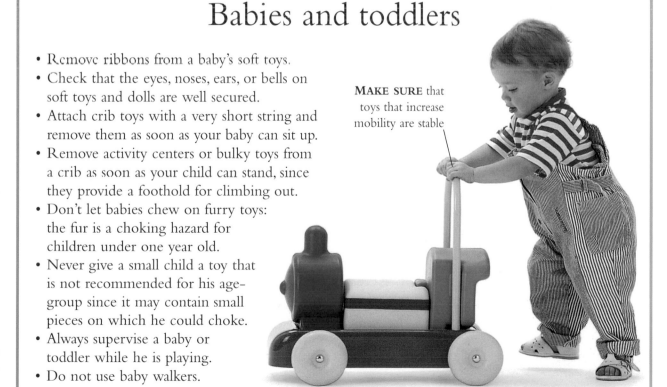

BEDROOMS

The cabinets and drawers in bedrooms are always exciting places for toddlers and young children. Make sure any potentially hazardous items are out of reach, because you may not always know when your child will decide to go exploring on his own.

Babies

CRIB

- Make sure the crib is deep enough to prevent your baby from climbing out – at least 26in (66cm) from the top of the mattress to the top of the crib.
- Bar spaces must be no more than 2⅜in (6cm) wide to prevent your baby's head from becoming trapped.

- The mattress must be the right size with no gap around the side; otherwise, the baby's head could get trapped between the side of the crib and the mattress. If two adult fingers can be placed between the mattress and the pad, the mattress should be replaced immediately.
- Do not use a pillow for a baby under one year: it could suffocate him. If you need to raise his head, put a pillow underneath the mattress.
- Use a sheet and woven blankets, rather than a comforter, until your baby is a year old. Your baby may get overheated or kick the comforter over his face and suffocate.
- Put your baby to sleep on his back with his feet at the foot of the crib to lessen the risk of crib death.
- Remove bumpers as soon as your baby can sit up because he could use them to climb out.
- Once he starts trying to climb out of the crib, transfer him to a bed. You can fit a bed guard at first, until he is used to the bed.

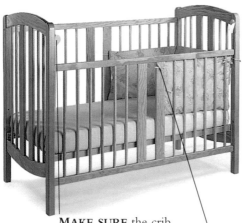

MAKE SURE the crib dropside has strong catches that your baby cannot open

ENSURE that bumpers have very short ties to prevent strangulation

CHANGING AREA

- Keep all changing equipment in one area, so that you never have to leave your baby alone. He will be safest on the floor, but if you have a changing table, remember that he might roll off if left for even a moment.
- Do not have shelves above the changing area in case something falls off.
- Keep mobiles out of his reach.

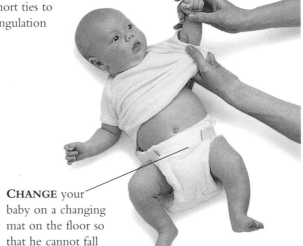

CHANGE your baby on a changing mat on the floor so that he cannot fall

118

Your child's room

BEDS

- Use a bed guard when your toddler first moves to a bed.
- Top bunk beds must have safety rails on both sides and any gaps in the railings or between the top of the mattress and the bottom of the safety rail should be less than 3½in (9cm).
- A top bunk is not recommended for children under the age of six.
- Never let young children play on the top bunk.
- Remove toys from the floor by the bed at night.

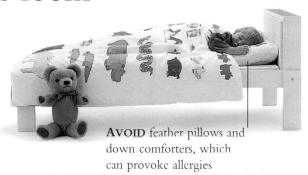

AVOID feather pillows and down comforters, which can provoke allergies

WINDOWS

Make sure your child can't climb out. Even if his room is on the first floor, he is in danger if he falls.

- Attach a safety latch, but make sure the window can be opened easily in the event of a fire.
- Try not to place a piece of furniture below a window – it may encourage your child to climb up.

TOYS (see p. 117).

- Try to keep toys with small pieces separate from others, so that you can easily remove them and put them out of reach for a while if your child is sharing a room with a toddler, or if you have young visitors.

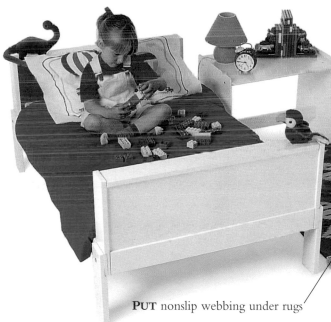

PUT nonslip webbing under rugs

Your room

- **Medicines and pills** Do not keep them beside your bed or on a dressing table. Put them out of sight and out of reach.
- **Scissors and sewing equipment** Keep these in a drawer or cabinet where your child cannot reach them.
- **Perfume, hairspray, and makeup** These can be harmful if sprayed or rubbed in the eyes, or drunk, so keep them out of reach or in a drawer with a safety catch.
- **China cups and glasses** Never leave a china cup or a glass on the floor by your bed. If your child is sleeping in your bed at night and rolls out onto the cup or the glass, he could have a serious accident.

BATHROOM

Your child may be at risk from falls, drowning, or poisoning in the bathroom. Keep the bathroom door shut at all times to discourage him from going in. On the inside of the door, fix the bolt high up to prevent a small child from locking himself in.

SHOWER
- Keep a constant check on the temperature of the water.
- Use nonslip mats in the shower and on the bathroom floor.
- Glass shower doors should be made of tempered safety glass or laminated glass.

BATH
- Always check the temperature of the water before your child gets in. A young child can be badly scalded by hot bathwater.
- Use nonslip mats in the bathtub and on the floor by the bathtub.
- Never leave a young child or baby alone in the bath. A baby can drown in just 1in (2.5cm) of water. If you need to answer the doorbell or telephone, take your child.

CABINETS
- Store bathroom chemicals and other potential poisons, such as toilet cleaners and bleach, out of reach in a cabinet with a safety catch.
- Keep other hazards, such as makeup, aftershave, razors, nail scissors, and any medicines or glass containers, out of reach in a locked medicine cabinet.

TOILET
- Use a special child toilet seat adaptor and step for toddlers, so that they can keep their balance more easily and feel more secure.
- Keep the toilet seat closed.
- Don't use block toilet cleaners that a small child could pull out and chew.
- Never mix toilet cleaners with bleach because this can give off toxic fumes.
- If your toddler uses a potty, keep it clean, but never leave bleach or cleaning agents inside it.

BATHE him away from the tap end

NEVER leave your child unattended in the bath

USE a nonslip mat in the bath

120

GARDEN

Your garden can be a safe and interesting place for your children to play. Children will find their own corners to play in but you should remove obvious hazards:

- Clear away any rubbish or rubble.
- Check garden furniture or play equipment regularly to make sure that it is stable, safe, and sited over a soft surface, such as grass.
- Keep pets out of areas where children play.
- Make sure paving is even and remove moss: children may easily trip or slip.
- Lock gates that lead out of the garden and make sure fences are secure.

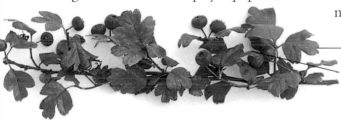

WARN your child not to eat berries or leaves

PLANTS

Many plants are poisonous if eaten and digested in large quantities. Small pieces, or one or two berries, may not be fatal, but may cause some discomfort and stomach upset.

- Tell your child about the dangers of eating berries, and keep babies and toddlers away from them.
- Remove plants that you know to be poisonous, such as deadly nightshade, laburnum, and toadstools.
- Cut back any prickly plants, such as roses, brambles, and holly – they can give nasty scratches, especially to the eyes.

SUPERVISE your toddler at all times. Check that he is playing in a clean, safe area with safe toys

SHEDS

These are exciting dens for children.

- If your shed is full of gardening equipment or tools, tell your child that it is out of bounds and keep it locked.
- Put any chemicals, such as weedkiller, slug pellets, and insecticides, out of reach.

PONDS, WADING POOLS, AND WATER BARRELS

Children are in danger if they slip and fall, even in shallow water.

- Never leave children unattended when they are playing in, or near, water.
- Cover ponds, water barrels, and empty trash cans that collect rainwater.
- Always empty out a wading pool when your children have finished playing in it, and turn it upside down in case it rains.

GARDENING

- Don't apply chemicals when children will be playing in the garden.
- Don't mow the lawn while children are close by, since stone chips may be dislodged and fly up into their eyes.
- Put away all garden tools when you have finished using them.

121

OUT AND AROUND

After the home, most accidents to children occur on the street. Teach your child the rules of the road from an early age, reminding him to stay alert for traffic and to cross in a safe place. It takes a long time for children to develop a true road sense.

AS A GENERAL GUIDE
- Three-year-olds can learn that the pavement is safe and the road is dangerous.
- Five-year-olds can learn how to cross the road, but they are still not able to put this knowledge into practice on their own.
- Eight-year-olds can cross quiet streets on their own, but are not yet able to judge the speed and distance of traffic.
- Twelve-year-olds can judge the speed of an oncoming car, but are still easily distracted by friends.

IN THE STREET
Whenever you are out with your child, show him how to be aware of his own safety.
- Use reins or a wrist strap for a toddler, to keep him from running off.
- Hold a young child's hand when you are near the road, or waiting to cross.
- Teach your child by your example and always find a safe place to cross. This may be:

> ▲ *A cross walk. Wait until traffic is clear. Point with your finger. When traffic stops, you and your child may cross the street.*
>
> ▲ *A traffic light. Encourage your child to press the button and tell him to wait until the traffic has stopped.*
>
> ▲ *An underpass.*
>
> ▲ *A footbridge or overpass.*
>
> ▲ *A corner at an intersection.*

Crossing the road

Teach your child the rules of the road:

▲ *Find a safe place to cross, then stop.*

▲ *Stand on the pavement, near the curb.*

▲ *Look all around for traffic, and listen.*

▲ *If traffic is coming, let it pass.*

▲ *When there is no traffic near, walk straight across the road.*

▲ *Keep looking and listening for traffic while you cross.*

BIKES
- Children younger than 10 years old should not bicycle on roads without adult supervision.
- Arrange for your child to have bicycle training before he starts on the roads.
- Make sure your child can be seen when he's riding his bike – with bright fluorescent colors by day and reflectors on his clothes and bike by night. He should always wear an approved helmet to protect his head.

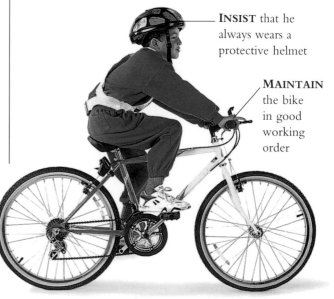

INSIST that he always wears a protective helmet

MAINTAIN the bike in good working order

PLAYING

What may seem common sense to you is not always obvious to children.

- Teach your child the dangers of playing in open areas, such as roads, construction sites, and quarries.
- Tell your child not to play in the street, or on a pavement near the curb.
- Tell him that he must never chase a ball, a pet, or another child into the road.
- Tell him not to try to cross the road from between two closely parked cars.

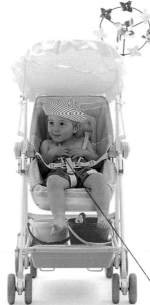

STROLLERS AND CARRIAGES

- Never push a stroller or carriage out into the traffic – pull it to one side and check whether it is safe to cross. Remember that a stroller sticks out in front of you by at least 3ft (1m).
- When you park a stroller or carriage, put on the brakes and point it away from traffic.
- Never tie your dog to the stroller.
- Never leave a baby unattended.

HARNESS your baby into his stroller

In the playground

Playgrounds should comply with safety standards and recommendations.

- The play area must be safely fenced off, away from roads.
- There should be a soft, even surface, such as bark chips or rubber tiles, around equipment.
- Slides should be no higher than 8ft (2.4m) and preferably constructed on an earth mound to break any falls.
- Roundabouts should be low, with a smooth surface, designed so that children can't get their feet stuck underneath.
- Jungle gyms or bars should be no higher than 8ft (2.4m), be completely stable, and built over sand or a very soft surface to break falls.
- There should be a clearly defined area for toddlers and young children, away from more boisterous older children.
- There should be someone to contact if equipment is faulty.
- Dogs must not be allowed inside playgrounds.
- Children should always be supervised by a responsible adult.

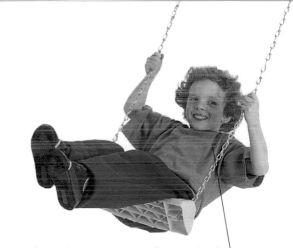

CHECK that swings are set apart from main play equipment, or fenced off, to prevent children from running in front of, or behind, them

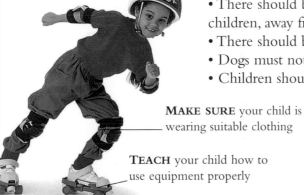

MAKE SURE your child is wearing suitable clothing

TEACH your child how to use equipment properly

STRANGERS *Remind your child of the dangers of talking to strangers. Have a code word that a friend can use if meeting your child. Tell your child not to go with anybody unless they use the code.*

GARAGE & CAR SAFETY

GARAGE

- Keep the garage locked and discourage your child from going in there.
- Keep equipment, chemicals, or tools out of your child's reach and locked away, if possible.
- Make sure you know where your child is when you are driving into, or out of, the garage.
- If you keep a freezer in the garage, it should be locked at all times.

CAR

- Never leave a young child unattended in a car.
- Don't let your child play with the windows, whether manual or electric. Windows can trap a child's head or fingers.
- Remove the cigarette lighter.
- Watch out for your child's fingers when you shut the doors.
- Use child locks on rear doors until your child is at least six years old.
- Teach your child to get out of the car on the curb side.
- If your child is helping you as you wash or clean up the car, make sure you have removed the keys from the ignition.

CAR SEATS

Always put your child into a special safety seat when you strap him into the car. Do not buy a second-hand car seat because some car seats are reconditioned after a crash and will not be safe. Choose the right seat for the weight and development of your child.

- **Babies** up to 22lb (10kg) – about 12 months – should travel in a rear-facing car seat. The baby is harnessed into the seat and the seat is held in place by the car seatbelts. The back seat is the safest place for all children to ride. Never place a rear-facing car seat in the front passenger seat if there is a passenger-side airbag because the impact of an airbag inflating could cause your baby serious head or neck injuries.
- Never carry a baby on your lap, or inside your own seatbelt: he would be crushed in a crash.
- **Older babies and toddlers**, up to 40lb (18kg), need a convertible car seat in the back. Some of these seats have an integral harness for the child that fits over his shoulders and between his legs. These seats are kept in place by the adult seat belt, or by straps that you can fix into the car. Other seats use the adult belt to hold both the child and the seat into the car.
- **Primary school children** should travel in a booster seat. Without it, adult seat belts are neither comfortable nor safe: the shoulder part cuts across the child's neck, and the lap strap lies across his stomach. In a crash, the lap strap can damage a child's liver or spleen. A booster seat raises a young child so the shoulder part lies across his upper chest and the lap strap lies across his hips. A lap strap on its own is not sufficient since it does not restrain the child's upper body.

FIT a convertible car seat for maximum protection

124

INDEX

127

Acknowledgments

ORIGINAL US EDITION
Project Editor Caroline Greene; **US Editor** Jill Hamilton;
Senior Art Editor Jane Bull; **Managing Editor** Jemima
Dunne; **Managing Art Editor** Tina Vaughan; **DTP
Designer** Karen Ruane; **Production** Maryann Rogers;
Photography Andy Crawford, Steve Gorton

Dorling Kindersley would like to thank:
Charlotte Stark and Dr. Mike Hayes of the Child Accident
Prevention Trust for reviewing *Safety In and Around the
Home*; Hilary Bird for the index; the following for
modeling:
Children Aleena Awan, Navaz Awan, Amy Davies,
Thomas Davies, James Dow, Kyla Edwards, Austin Enil,
Lia Foa, Maya Foa, Kashi Gorton, Emily Gorton, Thomas
Greene, Alexander Harrison, Rupert Harrison, Ben
Harrison, Jessica Harris-Voss, Jake Hutton, Rosemary
Kaloki, Winnie Kaloki, Ella Kaye, Maddy Kaye, Jade
Lamb, Emily Leney, Daniel Lord, Harriet Lord, Ailsa
McCaughrean, Fiona Maine, Tom Maine, Maija Marsh,

Oliver Metcalf, Eloise Morgan, Tom Razazan, Jimmy
Razazan, Georgia Ritter, Rebecca Sharples, Ben Sharples,
Thomas Sharples, Ben Walker, Robyn Walker, Amy Beth
Walton Evans, Hanna Warren-Green, Simon Weekes,
Joseph Weir, Lily Ziegler
Adults Shaila Awan, Claire le Bas, Joanna Benwell,
Georgina Davies, Marion Davies, Sophie Dow, Tina
Edwards, Rachel Fitchett, Emma Foa, Caroline Greene,
Susan Harrison, Victoria Harrison, Julia Harris-Voss, Emma
Hutton, Helga Lien Evans, Sylvie Jordan, Jane Kaloki, David
Kaye, Louise Kaye, Philip Lord, Geraldine McCaughrean,
Diana Maine, Brian Marsh, Jonathan Metcalf, Francoise
Morgan, Hossein Razazan, Angela Sharples, John Sharples,
Miranda Tunbridge, Vanessa Walker, Catherine Warren-
Green, Toni Weekes, Robert Ziegler

Makeup: Wendy Holmes, Pebbles, Geoff Portas
Additional photographs
Dave King, Ray Mollers, Suzannah Price, Dave Rudkin,
Steve Shott

EMERGENCY TELEPHONE NUMBERS

> **IN AN EMERGENCY DIAL 911 OR YOUR LOCAL EMERGENCY NUMBER. ASK FOR THE POLICE, AMBULANCE OR FIRE DEPARTMENT**

DOCTOR
Name: _____
Address: _____
_____
Telephone: _____
Office Hours: _____

POISON CONTROL CENTER
1-800-268-9017 or your local Poison Control Center number

DENTIST
Name: _____
Address: _____
_____
Telephone: _____
Office Hours: _____

HOSPITAL EMERGENCY DEPARTMENT
Address: _____
_____
Telephone: _____

EMERGENCY MEDICAL SERVICE (EMS)
Telephone: _____

LATE NIGHT PHARMACY
Address: _____
_____
Telephone: _____

LOCAL POLICE STATION
Address: _____
_____
Telephone: _____

GAS EMERGENCY SERVICE
Telephone: _____

ELECTRICITY EMERGENCY SERVICE
Telephone: _____

WATER EMERGENCY SERVICE
Telephone: _____

TAXI
Telephone: _____

IN CASE OF AN EMERGENCY PLEASE CALL: _____
_____

First Aid Training

First aid classes for all ages are offered by St. John Ambulance Canada and the Canadian Red Cross.
For further information, check the web sites of these organizations or get in touch with the local branch headquarters.